STRATEGIC PLANNING IN HEALTH CARE

A Guide for Board Members

Ellen F. Gold
and Kevin C. N

with a finance primer
by Jonathan G. Weaver

Ernst & Young LLP

AHA books are published by American Hospital Publishing, Inc.,
an American Hospital Association company

This publication is designed to provide accurate and authoritative information in regard to the subject matter covered. It is sold with the understanding that neither the authors nor the publisher is engaged in rendering legal, accounting, or other professional service. If legal advice or other expert assistance is required, the services of a competent professional person should be sought.

The views expressed in this publication are strictly those of the authors and do not necessarily represent official positions of the American Hospital Association.

Library of Congress Cataloging-in-Publication Data
Goldman, Ellen F.
     Strategic planning in health care: a guide for board members /
    Ellen F. Goldman, Kevin C. Nolan.
        p. cm.
    Includes bibliographical references.
    ISBN 1-55648-127-6
     1. Hospitals—Business management.   2. Hospital trustees.
  3. Strategic planning.   I. Nolan, Kevin C.   II. Title.
    [DNLM: 1. Hospital Planning—organization & administration—United
  States.   2. Planning Techniques.   3. Governing Board. WX 140 G619s
  1994]
  RA971.3.G57 1994
  362.1'068—dc20
  DNLM/DLC
  for Library of Congress   94-33244
                                          CIP

Catalog no. 196130

©1994 by American Hospital Publishing, Inc.,
an American Hospital Association company

Printed in the USA

AHA is a service mark of the American Hospital Association used under license by American Hospital Publishing, Inc.

Text set in Sabon
5M—12/94—0385

Richard Hill, Acquisitions/Development Editor
Lee Benaka, Production Editor
Peggy DuMais, Production Coordinator
Luke Smith, Cover Designer
Marcia Bottoms, Books Division Assistant Director
Brian Schenk, Books Division Director

Dedication

This book is dedicated to the clients with whom we have worked to shape a better health care system.

Contents

List of Figures and Tables

About the Authors

Ellen F. Goldman is a partner in Ernst & Young's health care strategic planning and marketing practice based in Washington, D.C. Ms. Goldman has over 16 years of experience in health care planning and marketing, both as a corporate director of a vertically integrated health care system and as a consultant to general and specialty hospitals, health care systems, physician practices, ambulatory care centers, nursing homes, home health agencies, and health-related organizations. She has conducted over 250 client engagements throughout the United States in the areas of strategic planning, marketing, market research, business planning, mergers and acquisitions, organization and governance, strategic operations planning, managed care, and network formation. Ms. Goldman has published over 20 articles on health care planning and marketing topics and holds board positions with the Alliance for Healthcare Strategy and Marketing and the American Association of Healthcare Consultants. She holds a bachelor's degree in economics and community health from Tufts University, Medford, Massachusetts, and a master's degree in business administration from the University of Pittsburgh.

Kevin C. Nolan is a partner in the strategy and marketing group of Ernst & Young's health care consulting practice. During his more than 15 years with Ernst & Young, Mr. Nolan has conducted over 300 strategic planning and marketing engagements for community hospitals, academic medical centers, multihospital systems, physician groups, long-term care providers, home health agencies, specialty facilities, and health care manufacturers and suppliers located throughout the United States. He has written several articles on strategic planning and is a frequent speaker at state and national meetings. Mr. Nolan received a bachelor's degree in government from the University of Notre Dame, Notre Dame, Indiana, and a master of management degree in hospital and health services management from Northwestern University, Evanston, Illinois. He is a member of the American Association of Healthcare Consultants and the American College of Health Care Executives. Mr. Nolan also serves as an associate professor at Johns Hopkins University.

Jonathan G. Weaver is an audit partner in Ernst & Young's Louisville office. During his 13 years with Ernst & Young, Mr. Weaver has been the firm's national director of health care industry accounting and auditing services. He has been responsible for technical guidance and support, as well as professional development, for the firm's health care audit practice. Mr. Weaver has served a wide variety of health care providers, including not-for-profit community hospitals, publicly held multifacility companies, psychiatric hospitals, home health agencies, and long-term care facilities. Mr. Weaver, a certified public accountant, graduated with honors from the University of Texas at Austin and is a member of the Texas Society of Certified Public Accountants and an advanced member of the Healthcare Financial Management Association.

Preface

Health care strategic planning has undergone tremendous change in the past several decades, from the setting of simple objectives to the development of laborious five-year forecasts; from an emphasis on centralized (corporate) activities to a focus on decentralized (operating unit) activities; and from the performance of detailed, data-intensive exercises to the conducting of cathartic group processes. In today's complex, competitive, and changing world of health care, it is easy to ignore planning and merely respond to the crises at hand. Ultimately, though, a health care organization without a direction is like the proverbial ship without a course—sooner or later it founders on the rocks of hard times.

The authors of *Strategic Planning in Health Care: A Guide for Board Members* believe in the maxim "failing to plan is planning to fail." Constant change does not make planning impossible—it makes planning imperative. But to be effective, strategic planning in the 1990s and beyond must be performed with several fundamentally different goals in mind:

- Planning must foster strategic thinking as opposed to simple extrapolations of the past.
- Planning must be carried out with attention to content (information) as well as to the process and the participants.
- Planning must provide the organizational cohesion (via vision, strategies, and tactics) to integrate the activities of departments, programs, services, and operating units.

Strategic Planning in Health Care: A Guide for Board Members is not intended to be used as a how-to manual. Rather, it is meant to convey to members of the boards of health care organizations an overview of the strategic thinking, planning, and integration process and board members' roles and responsibilities in this process. It is recognized that the management of health care organizations is responsible for leading by initiating, designing, and supporting organizations' planning processes. However,

xi

the ability of board members to provide meaningful input and evaluate planning processes and their outcomes will be enhanced by greater familiarity with the concepts and tools discussed herein.

This book updates and combines the contents of two previous publications of American Hospital Publishing, Inc.: *A Guide to the Board's Role in Strategic Business Planning* (1988), by John Abendshien, and *A Guide to the Board's Role in Hospital Finance* (1987), by Charles M. Bley and Cynthia T. Shimko.

Acknowledgments

The authors wish to express their appreciation to several people at Ernst & Young LLP for their help during preparation of this book. In particular, the authors thank Emmanuel V. Orfanon, Charles M. Bley, and Jonathan G. Weaver for their guidance and encouragement in developing the book's concepts and outline. The authors also wish to thank Jonathan Weaver for his finance primer, Harvey J. Gitel for his assistance on the finance primer, and the professionals of the Washington D.C.-based Strategy and Marketing Group for their technical advice and input to the main text of the book.

Additionally, the authors wish to thank Richard Hill and Lee Benaka of American Hospital Publishing, Inc., for their developmental and editorial efforts.

Introduction

One of the most important but least understood responsibilities of hospital board members today is their role in organizational planning processes. Most board members know that health care organizations, like other complex organizations, must clearly define the nature of their business, create a guiding strategy for fulfilling their objectives, and follow an orderly plan for future business development. But questions often arise: What constitutes a sound planning process? What should a strategic plan encompass? How does strategy development relate to operational planning and budgeting processes? What are the respective roles and responsibilities of hospital board members and managers in the overall planning process?

Most hospital board members and top-level managers are familiar with the term *strategic plan*. The strategic plan establishes a health care organization's vision and overall direction for the near term (usually three to five years). Mention of a strategic plan often conjures up images of hefty documents laden with data and analyses of previous years that inevitably conclude with the articulation of broad, lofty goals for the future.

Such strategic plans are inappropriate for two reasons. First, health care entities are undergoing a major paradigm shift, changing from independent organizations that provide illness-focused episodic care to networks and systems of entities that deal with the health needs of populations over entire lifetimes. When strategic planners extrapolate future goals on the basis of historical data and analysis alone, they ignore this paradigm shift completely and risk the development of an outmoded strategic plan. The planning process must allow for creative and futuristic thinking. Second, goals set without regard to the practical realities of economic and organizational constraints stand little chance of being achieved. Financial, operational, and organizational considerations must be part of the planning process.

The underlying thesis of *Strategic Planning in Health Care: A Guide for Board Members* is that strategic planning, if it is to provide organizational vision and cohesion, must foster strategic thinking that centers on the future, not the past. Strategic planning must integrate financial, operational, and organizational issues and resources into a unified set of activities that can be realistically accomplished.

This book should enable members of the boards of health care organizations to better understand the strategic planning process and their role in the process. It is important to note that all board members, along with top-level managers, share the responsibility for establishing strategic direction, setting priorities, and monitoring actual results against planned outcomes over time. Initiating and performing planning tasks to achieve organizational goals can be delegated to committees or staff members, but the overall direction and development of an organization's strategy and strategic plan are inherently the responsibility of the board and top-level managers. *Strategic Planning in Health Care: A Guide for Board Members* contains information that will help board members fulfill this responsibility.

Because strategic plans are intended to establish an organization's near-term strategic direction and plan of development, the full strategic planning cycle usually will not need to be repeated more often than once every three years. However, the action plans that are prepared in conjunction with the strategic plan constitute the organization's agenda for change and development, and they should be monitored on a quarterly basis and reviewed and revised on at least an annual basis. Indeed, action plan review should be an integral part of a health care organization's operational, planning, and budgeting cycle.

Emphasizing strategic thinking and integration, the first chapter of this book examines current business challenges in the health care field. Chapter 2 provides an overview of the planning function in the context of health care organizations. An overview of the strategic planning process is provided in chapter 3, and chapters 4 through 7 each address major internal and external planning considerations. Chapters 8, 9, and 10 consider specific phases of the planning process, including the strategic assessment, the establishment of a vision and strategies for development, and the creation of an implementation plan for strategy execution.

To effectively address the financial considerations in planning, many board members will want to refer to the finance primer at the end of this book. This primer helps board members understand health care financial matters and clarifies their role in this complex area.

Chapter 1

The Changing Dynamics of Health Care

The health care field of the mid-1990s is the subject of intense public scrutiny and heated political debate centered on the issues of skyrocketing costs, increasing unaffordability of insurance, and quality of care. Proposals to reform the system abound at local, state, and national levels. In such a highly charged and chaotic environment, health care strategic planning becomes marginally more difficult and infinitely more critical. This chapter provides board members with an overview of the underlying forces shaping the delivery system as well as the changing dynamics of the health care field. This overview will help board members to more clearly understand the challenges facing health care organizations.

Delivery System Drivers

The health care delivery system in the United States is driven by four interrelated factors: demographics, technology, financing, and human resources. This section explores each of these drivers and their impact on the delivery system.

Demographics

One of the principal influences on the health care delivery system is the size and age composition of the U.S. population, and the two most influential population segments are the *elderly* (people 65 years of age and older) and the *baby boomers* (people born between 1945 and 1965). The elderly have a major impact on the delivery system in three ways:

1. They consume health care services at a rate two to three times higher than the population as a whole.
2. Their numbers are increasing at a rapid rate. The number of people age 65 and older will total almost 35 million by the year 2000. This num-

ber represents an increase of more than 100 percent over the number
of elderly people in 1960.[1]
3. The elderly represent a formidable political force, with very effective
   lobbying organizations and a much higher rate of participation in local, state, and national elections than the general population.

The combination of their need for services, their increase in numbers, and
their active participation in the political process means that the elderly
will have a major say in the shape of the future health care delivery system
and how health care resources are allocated.

Although the elderly are a key population segment, the baby boomers
will ultimately drive the shape, size, and service configuration of the future health care delivery system. The dominance of the baby boomers will
be primarily a function of their sheer numbers. According to the U.S.
Bureau of the Census, although the elderly population will increase by
slightly more than 3 million people between 1990 and 2000, the population aged 35 to 54 will jump by more than 18 million.[2]

As this expanding population hits middle age, its need for and interest in health care will rise accordingly. This increased need for and interest
in health care could galvanize the baby boomers toward more political
participation, particularly as they continue to build their families. The
impact of the growing baby boom population on health care organizations will be significant as the health care needs of aging baby boomers
shift from birthing, "body repair" (orthopedic and intestinal surgeries),
and behavioral health (addictions and mental health services) to services
associated with more chronic and complex health threats such as cancer,
heart disease, and cerebrovascular disease.

Technology

Technology is a second determinant of the health care delivery system,
and the technological changes occurring in health care are even more profound than the demographic shifts described in the preceding section.
Among the major changes that board members must address are the dif-
fusion of technology (and the subsequent impact on cost and quality of
care) and the advances in medical technology (medical and surgical procedures, equipment, diagnostic tests, and drugs). Many of the technologies being introduced into community hospitals provide substantial benefits to patients, including improved outcomes, shorter inpatient stays,
delivery of care at alternative sites, and less-invasive procedures. In many
cases, this new technology also reduces the cost of care. However, it can
be argued that utilization of technology, as opposed to the actual capital
investment, contributes to increased national health care spending; never-

theless, the correlation between volume of procedures or tests and quality of care has been demonstrated conclusively in the medical literature.

Although advances in technology have produced additional benefits (and costs) to the health care system, these benefits have been largely incremental in nature. Future technological advances promise to bring a great deal of change and controversy to the health care field. In a two-part article on the reshaping of health care, futurist Jeff C. Goldsmith makes a compelling case that advances in predictive genetics and immunology will shatter the traditional paradigm of diagnosis and treatment and replace it with "one of prediction and early-stage management of illness, rendering much of our current armada of diagnostic and curative technologies obsolete."[3] Goldsmith notes that the American health care system has been organized to combat life-threatening acute illnesses, typically the result of infections born through foreign agents such as bacteria, viruses, or other parasites.

Advances in public health and medical science, combined with the aging of the population noted previously, have shifted the leading causes of death from infectious diseases to noninfectious and chronic diseases. Because chronic illnesses (those correlated with the aging process) have become America's leading health problem, board members of health care organizations need to replace their traditional view of health care with a new paradigm. This new paradigm will irreversibly and radically alter the notion of what health care is, where and when health care is rendered, and how health care is financed. This paradigm shift, fueled in part by the groundbreaking cooperative research being conducted by geneticists worldwide (the Human Genome Project), is inspired by the coming compression of major illnesses into shorter time spans at the end of life, as opposed to current illnesses that stretch out over several years and even decades. In addition, as Goldsmith argues, "To the extent that illness becomes predictable and manageable, our passive, reactive approach to financing and delivering care must give way to a proactive approach that implicates the patient, family, and society in appropriate measure in both the avoidance and ultimate financing of care."[4]

Financing

In terms of financing, another driving force in the health care delivery system, the health care field is undergoing a transfer of economic risk from the traditional buyers of health care services (governments, employers, and insurance companies) to the providers and consumers of health care. This phenomenon of risk transfer is resulting in a fundamental realignment of physician compensation, insurance payment methodologies, and patient cost sharing.

Physician Compensation

In terms of physician compensation, the traditional fee-for-service arrangement in which a patient or a patient's insurer paid separate charges for each office visit and procedure performed is giving way to arrangements in which physicians are salaried employees of health plans or are paid a flat fee per patient per month (known as *capitation*). In addition, some health plans reward physicians for keeping the cost of patient care down and drop those who fail to keep expenses in line. As a result of these changes in physician compensation, a system that used to provide a financial incentive to physicians to provide as much care as possible now encourages and rewards physicians who provide as little care as possible in appropriately meeting health care needs.

Insurance Payment Methodologies

Insurance payment methodologies are also changing substantially, shifting the economic risk of over- or underutilization of services from insurers to providers. As was the case with physicians, hospitals used to be reimbursed for the services they provided on a fee-for-service basis, a system that created an economic incentive for hospitals to maximize their "production." Now, hospitals are at risk of not being compensated for the costs associated with providing more (or less) care than is appropriate. This new risk is causing a drastic reduction in hospitals' utilization rates as they strive to align their treatment patterns with their payments.

Patient Cost Sharing

Historically, employers have played a relatively passive role in the health care system by providing their employees with insurance coverage and paying health care bills. However, recognizing that employee health care benefits are a business expense that must be managed like any other business expense, employers (particularly large employers) have begun to demand better deals from physicians, hospitals, and insurance companies. In response to receiving favorable financial terms from providers and insurers, employers have become more active in channeling new employees to those entities. Additionally, employers have begun to require that their employees bear more of the cost burden associated with the business expense of health care benefits. Insurance policies that paid 100 percent of all medical charges have been replaced with plans that require employees to pay increasingly higher copayments and/or deductibles. This shifting of economic burden and risk to the patient has reduced total utilization of health care services and shifted the timing of elective services to later in the employees' benefit year (after deductibles have been met).

Human Resources

The fourth driver of the health care delivery system is human resources. Health care has always been, and will almost certainly continue to be, a people-oriented business. At its core, health care is people helping other people; it is the laying on of hands (and, increasingly, technology) to help comfort and heal. However, it appears that demographic and sociological changes may combine to create a shortage of people to perform the laying on of hands (and technology). Specifically, U.S. demographic projections show virtually no growth in the number of people under the age of 24 through the year 2000 and a 7-million-person decline in the number of people between the ages of 25 and 34 during the same period.[5] These two age-groups have traditionally represented the pool from which health care providers drew the vast majority of nurses, therapists, and technologists.

With no growth expected in these population cohorts, providers will face increased competition for such employees, not only from within the health care industry, but also from other industries. The impact of this competition will be twofold: First, the price of obtaining personnel will rise, reflecting high demand and limited supply. Second, health care providers (including hospitals, physician offices, and other health-related organizations) will employ techniques and technologies from other industries to meet staffing challenges. These techniques and technologies might include retraining older workers (à la McDonald's), recruiting nationally and internationally rather than locally and/or regionally, and implementing technologies designed to reduce the need for increasingly scarce types of employees, as banks have done through the use of automatic tellers.

Changes in Delivery System Structure

The delivery system drivers described in the preceding sections are changing the fundamental structure of the health care field, and, as a result, new paradigms and critical success factors are emerging. Among the major health care structural shifts are the development of provider networks, the formation of physician groups, the integration of physicians and hospitals, the growth of managed care, and the prospect of health care reform. Figure 1-1 summarizes current and near-term trends in the health care field.

Development of Networks

At the time of this writing, about 60 percent of all hospitals in the United States were affiliated with formal multihospital systems. Only about 14 percent of hospitals participated in such systems during the 1980s, but

Figure 1-1. Current and Near-Term Trends in Health Care

	Now	Soon to Be
Structure	Independent providers and small systems ⟶	Large systems and networks
	Solo and small group practices independent of hospitals ⟶	Large groups integrated with hospital systems
	Providers separate from insurers ⟶	Integrated financing and delivery
Process	Illness-focused, episodic care ⟶	Health-status–focused care
Outcome	Emphasis on market share ⟶	Emphasis on covered lives
	Quality control through peer review ⟶	Quality control through outcome measurement

during the past few years the level of participation in hospital systems has increased exponentially.[6,7] This move toward affiliation represents a profound transformation in the underlying structure of the health care delivery system. Furthermore, the vast majority of hospitals, whether they are already part of a health care system or not, are aggressively exploring the possibility of establishing some type of partnership or alliance with other providers. These partnerships, alliances, and networks tend to be local or regional in scope and are primarily designed to deal with managed care organizations and new forms of payment, such as direct contracts or capitation. This affiliation trend is evident in virtually every health care marketplace and shows no signs of abating.

Formation of Group Practices

In addition to the affiliation of hospital providers, another fundamental shift in the structure of the health care field involves the movement of physicians into group practices and away from traditional solo practices or small single-specialty groups. The percentage of physicians who practice as part of a group is approaching 50 percent, which is up from less than 30 percent in the early 1980s.[8] Not only are physicians joining groups, but the size of these groups is increasing steadily as well, with a mean physician group size of almost 12 physicians.[9] Additionally, one of the fastest growing segments of group practice is physician groups with more than 100 physicians. This trend toward physician–physician integration shows no signs of slowing down and will almost certainly increase due to economic pressures and lifestyle considerations. For example, many primary care physicians in solo practice are experiencing overhead rates of greater than 50 percent (and growing), and recent surveys of physicians completing their training have revealed that less than 10 percent are interested in going into solo practice.[10]

Integration of Hospitals and Physicians

A third change in the health care delivery system structure is the evolution of hospital–physician relationships. Market forces are driving hospitals and physicians to reassess the traditional hospital–physician relationship model and to develop new, more closely integrated models and arrangements. These new arrangements unite physicians and hospitals through a structure (or structures) responsive to managed care and direct contracting forces and provide physicians with practice enhancement and management assistance.

A national survey of hospital chief executive officers, conducted by Ernst & Young in 1993, indicated that more than 20 percent of all hospitals had implemented some type of formal integration structure, an increase from the previous year, when less than 13 percent of hospitals had implemented formal integration. More than 75 percent of the CEOs surveyed indicated that they intended to develop such an integration structure if they did not already have one or develop an additional structure if they did already have one.[11] A key factor in successful hospital–physician integration efforts is the development of integrated structures in light of market factors and internal goals.

Growth of Managed Care

Perhaps one of the most significant changes affecting the structure of the health care field is the shift away from traditional forms of insurance toward managed care. Specifically, the number of Americans enrolled in indemnity insurance plans dropped from almost 9 in 10 in the early 1980s to less than 1 in 3 as of this writing. The number of people enrolled in managed care plans (health maintenance organizations and preferred provider organizations) is nearing 130 million, or about one-half of the population of the United States.[12,13,14] This growth of managed care from its status as an alternative system to the prevalent health care payment mode means that providers must decide *how* they should participate in managed care plans, as opposed to simply whether they should participate.

Potential Impact of Health Care Reform

Another issue to be considered in assessing the changing fundamental structure of health care is the potential impact of health care reform on the field and on the changes described in the preceding sections. The central issue of health care reform is whether any of the reform proposals will fundamentally change health care trends or create new ones. In reviewing the major health care reform proposals that have been debated in Congress during the past few years, a number of common themes emerge:

- Encouraging or requiring the development of integrated provider networks that offer a continuum of services to defined populations
- Establishing a payment mechanism that results in the increased assumption of risk by providers
- Mandating "universal" insurance coverage and a defined set of core benefits with guaranteed renewal for all legal residents
- Creating health insurance purchasing groups for individuals and small business owners
- Forcing provider networks to compete for patients on the basis of demonstrated outcomes and cost of services

These reform themes are entirely consistent with general trends in the health care field. In many areas of the country, the health care market is already reforming itself, and the adoption of formal legislation would simply codify changes already taking place. Therefore, the prospect of health care reform legislation (at either the national or local level) will serve to further accelerate the delivery system drivers and the changing structure of the health care field.

Implications for Providers

The fundamental restructuring of the health care field that is occurring as a result of the changing dynamics of health care will affect providers considerably. In assessing the implications of the changing dynamics of health care for providers, four areas of potential impact can be identified: geographic orientation, service scope, financial incentives, and organizational development.

Geographic Orientation

Health care, like politics, is local. Hence, the future state of health care will be locally based, with delivery systems built around regional networks of providers serving "natural" market or trade areas. Although the ultimate number of regional networks is impossible to predict, it does seem clear that the future health care delivery system will be oriented around large, tightly integrated systems of providers. The vast majority of providers will be a part of one (and possibly more) of these networks. Only those providers who are geographically isolated or whose services are unique will be able to remain independent. Similarly, small or geographically dispersed provider systems will seek to join (in some manner) larger, more geographically concentrated systems. All of these new systems will function more as true systems than do many of the current multihospital groups, which tend to operate more as loose confederations than as fully integrated systems with shared values and coordinated decision making and resource allocation.

Service Scope

The future health care delivery system will provide a coordinated, comprehensive continuum of health care services to a defined population group in the regional market area served by the system. This coordinated service complement will span the continuum from ambulatory care to institution-based care to home care.

Development of a service continuum will create at least four significant changes for many providers:

1. *The hospital will not necessarily be the center (or the owner) of the continuum.* In fact, in many cases, the hospital will represent only a minor component of the continuum, with much of the continuum's care rendered in noninstitutional settings and in the home as a result of technological advances.
2. *Many services of the continuum will be provided contractually rather than directly by the system.* The need to manage costs aggressively in order to be competitive will result in many systems determining that "buying" certain services from external providers is more cost-effective than "creating" those services internally.
3. *Some hospitals will likely drop marginal services from their service portfolios.* These services will be discontinued especially if they can be provided (or acquired) more cost-effectively elsewhere in the delivery system.
4. *The development of integrated systems and the establishment of contractual relationships will require new managerial skills, including system development and relationship management.* These skills are more externally focused and people intensive than the internally focused, financially oriented skill set that most hospital and health care managers have traditionally possessed.

Effectively addressing these changes in the future health care delivery system will help guarantee the success of providers.

Financial Incentives

One of the principal features of the future health care delivery system will be the continued push by payers (governments, businesses, and even individuals) to control the rate of increase in health care costs and at the same time maintain or even improve the quality of care provided. A focus on cost control and quality maintenance will shape the health care delivery system through the growth of capitation and a corresponding shift of risk to providers for the costs of over- and underutilization of services. This shift of risk to providers will provide a powerful incentive for them to provide care in the most appropriate and least costly setting.

In addition, as health care delivery systems become increasingly comprehensive in scope, both in terms of geography and service, they can bid on providing all health care (for a fixed fee) to large population groups such as unions, industrial workforces, or even entire cities. These comprehensive health care systems will not be paid by procedure, admission, or patient day but rather by person served. Being paid for "covered lives" dramatically changes providers' financial incentives. Instead of being driven to increase volumes of admissions or procedures, these capitated systems will strive to keep their covered populations as healthy as possible, thereby decreasing utilization.

Along with a shift in financial incentives from increasing service volumes to maintaining health, capitated systems will see a transformation of the economic engine that drives providers. Specifically, in a noncapitated system, the hospital is the economic engine, and a patient in one of its beds represents revenue. In a capitated system, a patient in one of its hospital beds represents cost. Therefore, the incentive for providers in capitated systems is to minimize the number of people in hospital beds by keeping them healthy. If people do become ill, providers will want to treat their conditions at the least costly sites, as appropriate.

Organizational Development

One central question concerning the future state of health care delivery relates to the issue of who or what will integrate care in the emerging regional delivery systems. Integrators will play the following critical roles in the formation and operation of provider networks:

- Creating local and regional delivery systems
- Developing financing mechanisms
- Allocating risk among network participants
- Negotiating with buyers
- Selecting network participants
- Developing infrastructure systems to link providers and support the network

Several entities have the potential to serve as the integrator. These players include existing hospital systems, insurance companies and health maintenance organizations, and large physician groups. Which of these entities emerges as the integrator will likely vary according to geographic region as a function of the relative degree of development and capabilities of each entity in its respective market.

Regardless of which entity ultimately plays the role of integrator, that entity will need to organize the service continuum in such a way as to minimize unnecessary duplication of services and achieve the lowest possible total cost per covered life. Some system components may incur additional costs at the unit level in order to optimize costs at the per-life level. Similarly, the integrator will be responsible for allocating resources (and financial risk) among the network participants, which will entail an entirely new set of managerial capabilities and relationships.

Summary

The industry drivers, structural changes, and implications described in this chapter are present, to a greater or lesser extent, in every health care market in the United States. Additionally, the pace and magnitude of changes affecting the health care industry are unlikely to moderate. No market or provider is so isolated or protected that it will not be affected by some, if not all, of these drivers, changes, and implications. Health care organizations therefore face a period of continuous turbulence in which change is the only constant.

In the increasingly chaotic and competitive health care marketplace, many health care executives and board members may question whether an organization will be able to plan at all, much less plan effectively. However, effective planning is possible in this complex and changing health care environment. In fact, the ultimate success of an organization depends on the ability of its board members and executives to develop a clear vision and shared understanding of where the organization needs to go, as well as a concisely articulated set of strategies and tactics to get the organization to that place. Constant change will make planning imperative. But to be effective, planning must undergo fundamental changes in how it is performed, who is involved in the process, what is included in the process, and how planning results are utilized.

References

1. U.S. Bureau of the Census. *Statistical Abstract of the United States: 1990.* 110th ed. Washington, DC: U.S. Government Printing Office, 1990, pp.16,18.

2. U.S. Bureau of the Census, pp. 16, 18.

3. Goldsmith, J. C. The reshaping of healthcare. *Healthcare Forum Journal* 35(5):19, May–June 1992.

4. Goldsmith, p. 27.

5. U.S. Bureau of the Census, pp. 16, 18.

6. American Hospital Association. *Directory of Multihospital Systems, Multistate Alliances, and Networks.* 4th ed. Chicago: AHA, 1982.

7. American Hospital Association. *American Hospital Association Guide to the Health Care Field.* Chicago: AHA, 1994.

8. American Medical Association. *Medical Groups in the U.S.: A Survey of Practice Characteristics.* Chicago: AMA, 1993.

9. American Medical Association.

10. Jolly, P., and Hudley, D. M., editors. *AAMC Data Book: Statistical Information Related to Medical Education.* Washington, DC: Association of American Medical Colleges, 1992.

11. Goldman, E., and Taulbee, P. *Hospital–Physician Integration: Results of a National Survey.* Alexandria, VA: Capitol, 1993.

12. Group Health Association of America. *1994 National Directory of HMOs.* Washington, DC: GHAA, 1994, p. 27.

13. Special report. *Employee Benefit Research Institute* 145:5, Jan. 1994.

14. HCFA Division of Medicaid Statistics. Statistical report on medical care: eligibles, recipients, payments, and services. *HCFA Report 2082,* July 1994, table 17.

Chapter 2

The Planning Function

Like other organizational functions, planning must change to reflect changing health care dynamics. The rapid changes of the 1990s call for shorter, more frequently revised action plans than were needed in previous years. The complex relationships that are forming among health care entities indicate the need for a broad planning focus and an openness to brokering and/or buying products and services, as opposed to creating those products and services internally. The more diverse a health care organization is, the more decentralized its planning process will be. Additionally, the participants in such a decentralized planning process will represent a wide spectrum of professions and functions.

The Purpose and Objectives of the Planning Function

Management has been generally described as the art of planning, leading, organizing, and controlling an organization's activities. The "job" of an organization's planning function can be further broken down to include the following seven responsibilities:

1. Designing and administering the corporate strategic planning process
2. Leading the development of corporate and business unit plans
3. Identifying and evaluating new business opportunities
4. Providing training and education related to planning
5. Conducting environmental scans and forecasts
6. Reconciling planning outcomes with capital and operational budgeting and facilities and human resource planning
7. Monitoring implementation actions

In summary, *planning* is a set of organizational activities aimed at figuring out what to do *and* how to do it. Planning should result in the following outcomes:

- *Directional guidance:* Determination of where the organization's attention should be focused
- *Assessments of the future:* Identification of what might reasonably be expected to occur as a result of planning
- *Resource allocation:* Specification of investment priorities
- *Performance standards:* Establishment of targets to facilitate control of planning goals

The Planning Function in Health Care Organizations

One of the few studies to gauge health care organizational planning practices, conducted by Ronald L. Zallocco and W. Benroy Joseph, reported that of the 13 activities generally considered to be part of strategic market planning (see figure 2-1), the three activities that fall under the heading of "environmental analysis" (that is, market analysis, competitive analysis, and general consumer surveys) are performed by fewer than half of the hospitals surveyed.[1] Specifically, 41 percent of hospitals surveyed report performing a market analysis, 45 percent report performing a competitive analysis, and 18 percent report conducting general consumer surveys. The percentage of hospitals that have completed environmental analyses is lower than the percentage of hospitals that have performed analyses of the other areas of strategic market planning. The only individual planning activity that received a lower completion ranking than environmental analysis was "budget allocation to planning," with only 27 percent of hospitals reporting that they had a formal planning budget. The two strategic market planning activities performed by the highest percentage of responding hospitals are identified as "existence of formal objectives" (90 percent) and "patient satisfaction surveys" (83 percent). From their data, Zallocco and Joseph conclude that "many hospitals set objectives and develop new programs without conducting a thorough and systematic assessment of their internal and external environments."[2]

Zallocco and Joseph also measured hospital administrators' satisfaction with their organizations' strategic market planning. They report a significant correlation between the level of satisfaction and two factors: (1) the level of planning maturity and (2) the extent of performance of planning activities. That is, administrators whose hospitals perform more planning activities with more sophistication are more satisfied with the planning results.

A tool developed by Ernst & Young to assess the quality of the plan-

Figure 2-1. Thirteen Typical Strategic Market Planning Activities

Environmental Analysis

1. Market analysis
2. Competitive analysis
3. General consumer surveys

Business Definition and Mission Statement

4. Existence of strategic marketing plan
5. Existence of formal business definition or mission

Objectives and Strategy Development

6. Existence of formal objectives
7. Formal new program development
8. Use of planning models in strategy development

Tactics

9. Advertising and promotion
10. Fund-raising programs

Budget and Control Mechanisms

11. Program evaluation and review
12. Patient satisfaction surveys
13. Budget allocation to planning

Source: Zallocco, R. L., and Joseph, W. B. Strategic market planning in hospitals: is it done? does it work? *Journal of Health Care Marketing* 11(1):5–11, Mar. 1991.

ning function in hospitals has produced findings similar to those of Zallocco and Joseph.[3] Applications thus far indicate that planning efforts rely heavily on historical data; however, projections and forecasts are infrequent, and few formal planning budgets exist. Other findings indicate that management education regarding planning is generally lacking and that planning interfaces poorly with the activities of the finance, facilities, and human resources departments. Satisfaction with the planning function is strong where written documents with measurable goals are produced.

It seems that planning is becoming so programmatic and pragmatic that some of the general tasks of the planning function are falling by the wayside. Additionally, the clear articulation of corporate strategies is in danger of being compromised. Program planning is a necessity, but it is not a starting point. Without a database of general market, competitor, and consumer information, planning for programs with immediate implementation schedules may lead to the following undesirable outcomes:

- *Opportunity costs:* The organization selects the wrong programs to implement.

- *Market saturation:* If thorough market analysis, which could provide a framework for service development and an understanding of how demand may be shifting among various services, is not performed, demand for the service may not materialize.
- *Unmet expectations:* If consumer and payer views, as well as how competing services differ from each other, are not considered when programs are developed, dissatisfaction with the service developed may result.

Moreover, without a clearly articulated vision and direction, the organization will vacillate among programs, unable to realize overall synergy.

The Impact of Change on the Planning Function

The trends and factors discussed in chapter 1 suggest that virtually all health care organizations—for-profit and not-for-profit—now assume business risk in much the same manner as other corporate and business enterprises. This assumption of risk has a direct effect on the need for, and the nature of, the organizational planning process. Recent changes in the health care field have affected organizational planning in at least three ways.

First, although many organizations formerly assigned organizational planning responsibility to staff planners, the relative importance of the planning function and the consequences of poor planning decisions are so great in the 1990s that neither board members nor top-level managers can afford to fully delegate the planning process. In particular, board members must realize that health care organizations are exposed to considerable business risk in today's environment and that the board has a fiduciary responsibility to ensure that sound business planning is exercised.

Second, organizational planning can no longer be a sporadic, ad hoc activity performed in response to specific project initiatives or immediate threats or concerns. Planning must be a continuous and ongoing process. It must be a discipline that ensures an orderly assessment of needs, opportunities, and risks, as well as a discipline that establishes business direction and resource allocation priorities within an economically sound framework.

Third, organizational planning has historically emphasized a service market focus. Although such a focus is still relevant, a much broader focus is required for today's planning process. Market and service information must be integrated with financial data and analyses. In addition, the plans themselves must clearly address capital requirements and organizational development needs.

Overall, the planning process must provide a framework for guiding all of the decisions made by the board and top-level management regarding strategic priorities, capital and operating budgets, and organizational development. This framework is, in effect, an evolving blueprint for the organization's agenda for change.

The Roles and Responsibilities of the Board and Management

Because the strategic planning process is critical to a health care organization's future direction and economic well-being, planning is by its very nature the joint responsibility of the organization's board members and senior managers. In the broadest sense, the board's responsibilities in the planning process are the following:

- Ensuring that sound planning policies and processes are in place
- Making policy decisions regarding overall strategic direction and corporate objectives
- Ensuring that the organization's strategic direction is consistent with its overall mission
- Reviewing and approving specific project initiatives and action plans to ensure consistency with the strategic direction
- Ensuring that the organization's financial and human resources are accessible and invested in a manner that will support the strategic direction
- Monitoring strategic plan implementation and organizational performance relative to the strategic plan

The planning responsibilities of the chief executive officer (CEO) and other top-level managers include the following:

- Designing and initiating the planning process and maintaining the organization's planning calendar
- Gathering data and performing analyses, as required, to support the planning process
- Assuming a leadership role in formulating an overall strategic direction and development objectives, subject to the board's review and approval
- Creating action plans in support of the strategic direction and updating those plans at least annually

- Developing investment criteria (consistent with the strategic plan) that provide a basis for rational, proactive decisions regarding the allocation of resources
- Developing management–board reporting mechanisms to provide continuous monitoring of plan implementation results
- Involving appropriate representatives from the board, management, medical staff, and other constituencies in the planning process

These two sets of responsibilities clearly indicate that the implementation and performance of strategic planning activities are principally the responsibility of the CEO and top-level managers. However, board members have a primary responsibility to ensure that planning is accomplished and, further, that the actions taken are consistent with the organization's overall strategy and objectives.

Medical staff members and other professional staff members should be afforded the opportunity to provide input in the strategic planning process. These individuals can provide valuable insights for identifying clinical strengths and weaknesses, program development priorities, and technological requirements. Such input is often provided by physicians who serve on the board or who are salaried members of the management team. In addition, input from individual physicians and clinical departments is often obtained through interviews and surveys, as discussed in chapter 8.

Many health care organizations create a planning committee consisting of board members, senior managers, and professional staff members to conduct and monitor strategic planning activities. In some organizations the executive committee of the board (or sometimes the entire board) fulfills these planning responsibilities. Regardless of how planning responsibilities are assigned within the organization, those who occupy positions of ultimate approval and decision-making authority must be closely involved in the planning process. Planning is not a responsibility that should be delegated to a lesser authority.

A question often arises about whether it is helpful to employ an outside consultant either to facilitate the strategic planning process or to act as an adviser. The answer to that question depends on a variety of factors, including the following:

- Whether the organization has previous planning experience and a well-defined approach to the planning process
- Whether critical or sensitive issues exist that require outside objectivity
- Whether management has enough time and expertise to make the process work

Outside advisers do add an important dimension of objectivity, and they are not encumbered by vested interests or personal agendas. In addition, outside advisers can provide a broad perspective on how global trends and events may potentially affect particular health care organizations.

Even when an outside consultant or facilitator is brought into the planning process, board members and top-level managers must remain actively involved. In many respects, the planning process itself is more important than the results of planning. Those responsible for plan development and execution must reach a consensus regarding the organization's position, strategic direction, and development priorities. This consensus, or "buy-in," is achievable only through the direct involvement of board members and top-level managers in the planning process.

Summary

Sweeping changes in the health care field have affected the nature of the organizational planning process and have raised it to a new level of importance. Although the health care field formerly focused on the expansion of services and facilities in a growth market, health care entities are now faced with changing demand patterns, price constraints, and intensified competition, all of which have affected planning requirements. Today's high-risk health care environment calls for a broad planning focus linking market, service, and financial analyses. Previously, planning was performed largely on an ad hoc, project-specific basis; today, planning must be performed continuously. In addition, because health care organizations face more risk in today's environment, board members and senior managers assume a greater responsibility for planning.

References

1. Zallocco, R. L., and Joseph, W. B. Strategic market planning in hospitals: is it done? does it work? *Journal of Health Care Marketing* 11(1):5–11, Mar. 1991.

2. Zallocco and Joseph, p. 8.

3. Goldman, E. F. *Checklist for Assessing the Quality of the Planning Function in Your Health Care Organization*. Washington, DC: Ernst & Young, 1989.

Chapter 3

Overview of the Strategic Planning Process

This chapter briefly describes the components of a sound strategic plan. In addition, this chapter discusses in general terms the three primary phases of the planning process (described in more detail in chapters 8 through 10) and lists the most common participants in the process and their respective roles. This overview chapter also sets the stage for chapters 4 through 7, which describe specific considerations in planning from the market, operational, financial, and organizational perspectives.

The Essential Components of a Strategic Plan

The components of a strategic plan vary depending on the organization's businesses, situation, issues, needs, and planning requirements. However, all strategic plans should have the essential components of vision, focal areas, strategies, action plans, and planning databases.

Vision

Every health care organization should have a clear definition of where it is headed, that is, what the organization will look like when it achieves its strategic plan. This vision should be more than a statement of mission, which is usually specific to the working goals of the organization and rarely directional. Vision focuses the organization on what it wants to be in terms of markets, services, technology, and delivery settings. The vision describes the entirety of the organization's future aspirations, well beyond the sum of the parts.

The difference between vision and mission can be clarified by considering the vision and mission of one well-known cancer center. The center's vision is "to unravel the mystery of cancer"; its mission, "to reduce the burden of human cancer," is more concrete.

Focal Areas

Achieving a health care organization's vision requires the identification of several focal areas, usually between four and eight broad categories of activities. In order to optimally focus attention, it is essential to limit the number of focal areas. Numerous focal areas may indicate an overly ambitious plan or reveal areas that can be combined for better synergy. Focal areas often relate to service development, physician integration, operational restructuring, and market relationships.

Each focal area should have two components. One is a developmental goal, usually presented as an action statement. The other component is an objective or target for measuring goal achievement. Objectives or targets are often set for the following areas:

- Market penetration
- Quality standards
- Operational effectiveness
- Profitability
- Return on investment

Strategies

Strategies must be formulated to specify exactly how the health care organization will fulfill its vision and attain the objectives that are part of the organization's focal areas. Focal areas indicate what needs to be done, and strategies delineate how that action will be carried out. For example, a focal area goal might be to improve the accessibility of primary care services to the local market. Strategies to achieve that goal might include (1) locating walk-in primary care centers in identified areas of opportunity in the community and (2) expanding on-site outpatient services and facilities for primary care. Collectively, focal areas and strategies provide health care organizations with a blueprint for achieving future development.

Focal area goals and strategies also provide a framework for evaluating the major decisions that the organization will face in the years ahead. Together with the objectives to be achieved, these two components address several important questions: What is needed? What is realistic and affordable? Does a proposed initiative meet strategic objectives as well as economic criteria? Such an evaluation framework expedites a health care organization's decision-making process. This framework also minimizes the risks and opportunity costs that are associated with making wrong decisions.

Action Plans

Action plans translate strategies into action steps, identify resource requirements, establish timetables, and assign responsibilities. They identify the tasks that need to be completed and set quarterly time frames as targets for implementation. Resource requirements in action plans are outlined at a high level and include capital, staffing, facility, and other organizational requirements.

Planning Database

Although it is not necessarily part of the written strategic plan, one result of the planning process is a planning database that can be periodically updated. This planning database, which would include market information, performance and competitor data, financial ratios, and so forth, can be used to compare actual performance to initial performance goals.

The Strategic Planning Process

In its simplest form, *strategic planning* can be defined as the process of strategy assessment, development, and implementation. During each of these three main steps, choices are made, actions are taken, and progress is measured. The manner in which an organization conducts its planning process varies according to the organization's operations and culture and the specific situations within the organization that are driving or inspiring the planning process. Certain planning activities, however, are essential and should be part of every organization's overall approach. These activities are discussed in the following sections and illustrated in figure 3-1.

Strategic Assessment

The strategic assessment includes an evaluation of the overall health care field, as well as the local health care market and the organization's position within the market. In addition to assessing health care market conditions and trends, an analysis of the market's competitive structure and a forecast of future structural changes are essential. The strategic assessment also includes an analysis of the organization's key characteristics (for example, operating and financial performance) in light of changing market structures. A base-case financial scenario assuming no significant change in the health care organization's strategic position is also developed.

Figure 3-1. The Strategic Planning Process

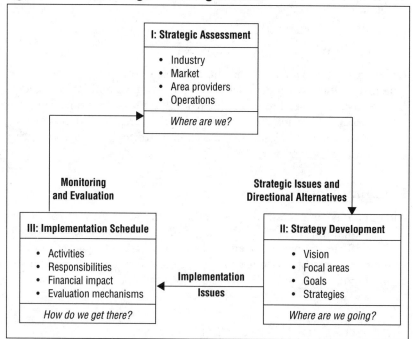

Strategy Development

The components of strategy development include evaluating alternative strategic directions for the organization, selecting the best course to follow, and crafting a statement of vision and related focal areas, goals, and strategies. Strategy development is generally a qualitative, process-oriented activity that requires creativity and challenges the information and forecasts prepared in the strategic assessment. The methods of strategy development are process oriented and vary considerably from organization to organization.

Implementation Schedule

The final step in the strategic planning process is to create explicit implementation/action plans that identify the tasks to be accomplished, the roles and responsibilities of key players, and the timetable for each program or project initiative. It is important to remember that the output of planning is not a plan; the output of planning is action.

Participants and Roles in Strategic Planning

The strategic planning roles and responsibilities of board members and top-level managers were defined in chapter 2. In determining who should participate in a health care organization's actual planning process, all of the organization's major constituents, as well as potential constituents, should be given consideration. These constituents include the following:

- *Members of the board of directors,* who have fiduciary and community responsibilities
- *Medical staff members,* who will need to integrate more closely with other providers
- *Management,* because the doers must be the planners
- *Employees,* because decisions affecting their jobs and performance need to be understood
- *Members of the community at large,* who utilize the organization's services
- *Health plans,* because of their increasing role in determining the health care delivery system
- *Employers in the business community,* because of their role as payers for services
- *Members of affiliated organizations,* who may depend on the organization for services or market share
- *Potential collaborators,* specifically, members of community organizations and other area providers who can help assess needs in order to avoid costly duplication of services

Each of the preceding groups should provide input and/or become involved in developing strategies through a participative process that is responsive to the health care organization's unique situation. The tendency to include every possible constituent must be balanced by the organization's time constraints, the resources committed to the planning process, the need for groups of manageable sizes, and the ability of participants to provide valuable input, address complex issues, and make decisions.

Summary

A health care organization's strategic plan should include a clear definition of the organization's vision, specific areas of focus and appropriate development objectives, strategies for accomplishing the vision, and action plans for the initiatives identified. The strategic planning process includes three steps: strategic assessment, strategy development, and implementation schedule development. The planning process and its participants will vary by organization, but planning decision makers should generally include medical staff members, payers (employers and health plans), management, and board members.

Chapter 4

Market Considerations in Planning

More than any other factor, the marketplace is driving change in the health care field. Regionalization, capitation, and collaboration are changing the market requirements related to each health care provider's services, size, and structure. To understand how marketplace forces will affect a health care organization, careful assessment of the market and thoughtful development of assumptions regarding the market's future state should be the cornerstones of the organization's strategic plan.

Market Definition

The definition of the market for health care services has typically been determined through analysis of patient origin. Although this method is helpful in painting a picture of the past, it is of less value in planning for future action. Patient origin does not equate with market share, and as such, areas of large population from which only a small portion of the market is loyal are often overemphasized. Patient origin is often related to the location of physician offices and may not reflect potential volume if additional resources were present in the community. Additionally, with payers directing more of the patient volume, arbitrary boundaries of "primary" and "secondary" services areas may be moot, and broader geographic definitions may be more accurate. With increasing consolidation and network development, markets that are regional in nature will be more relevant than those markets defined as local. Thus, the health care organization may use several different market definitions for analytical purposes.

The following information should be considered in determining the *broad market area* within which a health care organization exists:

- *Natural economic trade areas:* Metropolitan area zones, population patterns for major shopping and entertainment centers, and so forth

- *Current and proposed transportation systems:* Access enhancers (interstate highways, direct subway lines) and access barriers (rivers, mountains)
- *Employment patterns:* Locations of major employers of area residents and residences of area employees
- *Residential migration patterns:* Historical residential origin of the area's population (are people new to the area, did they migrate from the city, and so forth)
- *Proposed economic development:* The type of economic development plans that exist in an area, the magnitude of those plans, and the potential for those plans' success

Specific service draw areas are discussed later in this chapter under the heading "Market Size."

Market Structure

In order to understand the dynamics of current and future market behavior, health care organizations must consider four key elements of market structure. These four elements are degree of organization, degree of regulation, existence and profiles of area providers, and market potential.

Degree of Organization

Typically, hospitals, physicians, and payers have been separately and independently organized. However, in many areas of the country, economic pressures are fostering mergers, integration, and consolidation among these three parties. Such concentration will have a strong influence on where and how individuals gain access to health care services and how their care is paid for. The organization of the marketplace should be clearly tracked, and future organizational structures should be anticipated. Tracking of marketplace organization can be accomplished through analysis of the following characteristics:

- Number and size of purchasers
- Type of service arrangement (capitated, exclusive, preferred, episodic)
- Configuration and comprehensiveness of network participants
- Integration of purchasers and providers

Table 4-1 depicts a spectrum of market structures. It should be noted that each payer or provider group may be at a different point on the continuum.

Table 4-1. Market Structure Continuum

	Loose →		Consolidated
Payers:			
Employers	Independent employers	Employers eliminate plans to reduce administrative complexity	Health care purchasing cooperatives buy services; direct contracting increases
Insurers	Independent HMOs/PPOs; HMO penetration less than 30%; "managed indemnity"	Lead HMOs/PPOs achieve critical mass; selective contracting by major players; HMO penetration 30–50%	Shake out of weaker insurers; HMO penetration 50%+
Government	Government-managed Medicaid/Medicare programs	Optional enrollment of Medicaid/Medicare recipients into qualified managed care plans	Medicaid/Medicare population largely enrolled in managed care plans
Providers:			
Physicians	Solo and small group practices that are independent of hospitals	Development of large multispecialty and IPA groups; leading groups commit to managed care	Need for improved utilization and capital leads groups to seek hospital integration
Hospitals	Independent hospitals; weak hospital affiliations	Hospital affiliations/systems form; aggressive competition for physician group practices, efforts at physician integration	Consolidation eliminates redundant capacity; integrated delivery systems advance
Other	Independent long-term care, home care, freestanding ambulatory providers, and so forth	Consolidation of freestanding providers	Integration into health care delivery systems
Basis for purchasing	Encounter; cost of claim	Cost per covered life per health plan	Beneficiary health status; total health care cost
Basis of competition	Service, technology, relationships	Price	Price, outcomes

Degree of Regulation

Highly regulated health care markets represent barriers to new entrants and to existing providers attempting to develop new services or technologies. Additionally, some state and federal agencies are encouraging the use of health care providers that meet certain cost and/or quality standards.

Existence and Profiles of Area Providers

Other organizations providing health care services for the market area should be examined to gain insight into the relative strength of their market position and the market as a whole. Studies of other health care organizations should also assess their staying power and project the strategic requirements of initiatives that organizations in the market area might undertake. Specifically, a profile of other market-area providers should produce the following categories of useful information:

- *Service scope:* What types of services does each organization provide?
- *Technological breadth:* What is the range of technology offered by each organization?
- *Market position:* What is the respective market penetration (percentage of all patients served in the market) of each organization? How has that penetration changed, if at all, over the past three years or so?
- *Image:* What is the public's perception of each organization and its level of quality? How does the management and medical staff of the health care provider compiling the profile perceive other market providers?
- *Cost position:* How do published or contracted prices compare among the area's providers? To the extent that cost data are available, what are the relative costs per discharge for each organization?
- *Operating performance:* Given the available data, what are the respective profitability levels among other providers in the market area? What are the overall market trends concerning costs, revenues, and profitability?
- *Financial position and asset management:* What are the respective fund balances among area providers? What are their returns on assets? What is the average age of assets for each organization?

Figure 4-1 provides an example of a comparative profile of market-area providers that utilizes categories similar to those in the preceding list.

Market Potential

There are two reasons why it is critical to analyze health care market

Figure 4-1. Example of a Comparative Profile of Market-Area Providers for a Metropolitan Market

Indicator	Memorial	General	Carecor	Physicians' Medical Group	Community Health Plan	National HMO
Financial performance	3	1	1	2	1	1
Cost position	3	2	2	3	3	1
Market performance	2	1	1	3	1	2
Geographic location	3	3	1	2	1	1
Service growth	3	1	1	3	2	2
Diversification	3	1	3	3	2	1
Resource availability	3	1	1	3	1	1
Summary position	3	1	1	3	1	1

Note: Relative market strength is rated on a scale of 1 to 3, with 3 indicating a strong provider and 1 indicating a weak provider.

potential. First, projecting future aggregate service demand levels on a marketwide basis enables an organization to assess the potential effects that volume shifts may have on its business. Second, examining present and projected future demand on a case-specific or service-area basis makes it possible for an organization to identify unfulfilled service demands.

It is not the purpose of this book to provide an in-depth explanation of demand analyses and demand forecasting. However, the following basic principles should be mentioned:

- The total demand for health care services in any given market is finite, and total demand is declining for many inpatient services as length of stay is reduced and outpatient alternatives are developed.
- Forecasts should be projected for at least five years to fully take into account technological and service delivery advances.
- Multiple scenarios should be run on the basis of a range of demand assumptions.

Figure 4-2 illustrates inpatient bed need for a health care organization based on alternative scenarios of inpatient market demand according to changes in admission rates and length of stay. At a facility level, volume for all services should be projected, as shown in figure 4-3.

Figure 4-2. Sample Estimates of Inpatient Bed Need

Length of Stay (days)	Admissions per 1,000			
	110	100	90	80
7.0	1,241	1,128	1,015	902
5.5	975	886	798	709
3.5	620	564	508	451

Note: Based on a population of 500,000. Bed need assumes 85% occupancy.

Figure 4-3. Facility-Specific Service Requirements

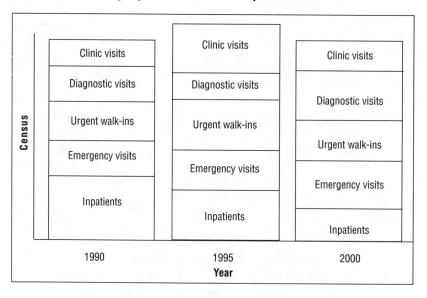

Market Channels

Knowing the market's structure will be of little value if relationships are not developed with the numerous market channels between a health care provider organization and its patients. These channels, which are illustrated in figure 4-4, include the following:

Figure 4-4. Market Channels

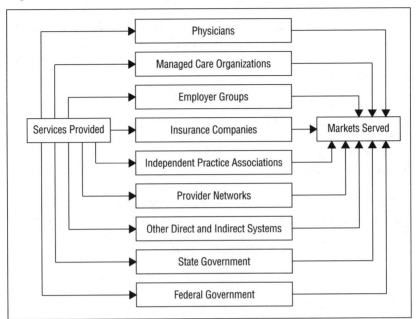

- Physicians and physician practice organizations
- Provider networks
- Employers
- Health plans
- Insurers
- Government entities

The nature and degree of contracting in the health care marketplace, whether the contracting is done with managed care plans, employers, or other entities, will affect where and how people decide to receive health care services. Such contracting arrangements will influence the flow of patients and health care dollars in markets where health plans have a high level of penetration and concentration and exert strong utilization control. Similarly, a high degree of employer concentration or business coalition activity in a market area will have a strong influence on where and how individuals obtain health care services, how individuals are treated, and how their care is paid for. Thus, it will be critically important for health care organizations to monitor insurance plans and employer and network activities. Each group's enrollment, utilization, plan coverage and terms, as well as potential changes in those areas, must be carefully tracked. These specifics will be essential to determining marketplace power shifts and crafting responsive organizational strategies.

Market Relationships

In addition to the provider networks that form important channels to the health care market, other types of provider and nonprovider relationships may be formed across the market for a variety of purposes, including the following:

- Continuum of care development
- Market coverage under contracting
- Service sharing and economies of scale
- Economic clout
- Community development

It is important to understand existing market relationships and assess their success and potential. Similarly, future market relationships should be anticipated, because they have the potential to change the structure of the marketplace and shift its balance of power.

Market Size

A health care facility's *market area*—the area from which it *could* draw patients if the appropriate channels and relationships discussed earlier in this chapter were in place—should be analyzed to understand how market characteristics may affect current and future demand for health care services. Such an analysis should consider transportation systems, economic development patterns, and migration patterns (all of which were discussed earlier in this chapter), as well as the following characteristics:

- *Population shifts:* Significant population increases or declines projected within the overall market area or within a portion of the market area can change health care utilization rates.
- *Age characteristics:* The need and demand for health care services can vary significantly among various age and sex cohorts. Health care needs are minimal for the pediatric population (0–14 years of age), but these needs increase for women of child-bearing age (15–44 years of age) and increase significantly for both sexes after age 45. The number of physician office visits, ambulatory encounters, and hospital patient days generated per 1,000 people is, on average, two to three times greater for people over age 65 than for the population as a whole.
- *Socioeconomic characteristics:* An understanding of the income char-

acteristics of a health care organization's market area can indicate service needs and opportunities and can also point out the economic risks associated with caring for the medically indigent. State-sponsored public aid programs provide some reimbursement for individuals below a specified income threshold. However, in some markets many individuals earn incomes that are too high to qualify for public aid but are insufficient to pay for all health care needs.

- *Vital statistics:* Determining the major causes of a market area's mortality, morbidity, and birth rates, as well as other public health statistics, can alert hospitals to health service needs and opportunities.

Patient draw areas will vary depending on the specific service under consideration. Outpatient services typically have much smaller draw areas than do inpatient facilities, as shown in figure 4-5.

Market Manpower Resources

An often-overlooked market component of the health care planning process is the human resources available in the marketplace. In addition to sizing the future market demand for health care services, boards must translate that demand into manpower, that is, how many physicians, nurses, allied health professionals, and support personnel are needed to meet the demand. These manpower requirements should then be compared to available community resources. Key considerations when making this comparison include the following:

- Recruitment and retention strategies
- Past recruitment and retention performance
- Appropriate use of allied health professionals
- Effects of managed care on manpower needs
- Cross-training potential
- Partnering opportunities in staffing, education, and training

Another important consideration in determining manpower supply is the organization of medical resources in the community. As noted earlier in this chapter, medical groups, through independent practice associations and other physician organizations, can become channels to the market, and hospitals should develop strategies to create relationships with them. Additionally, large group practices are often overlooked as competitors (or potential competitors) to hospitals, and their place in the community should also be analyzed.

Figure 4-5. Service Draw Areas

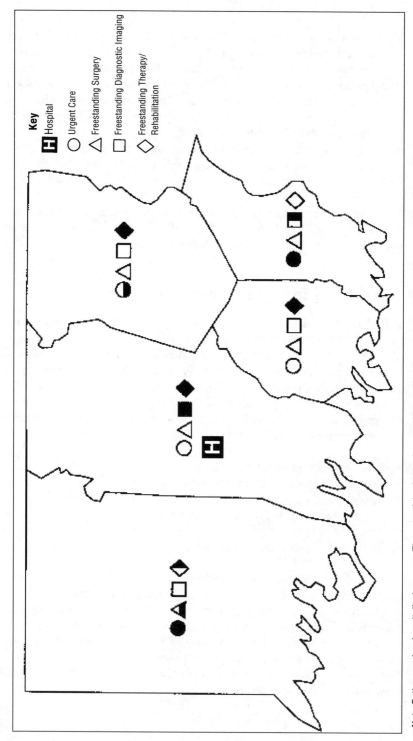

Note: Entire area is a hospital's draw area. The potential volumes in outpatient service draw areas are indicated by percentage of shape filled. Closed = high volume and open = low volume compared to current capacity in market.

Summary

Board members need to understand the structural and behavioral characteristics of the external marketplace, the capabilities and direction of other area providers, the major demands of the market, and the potential for future services to the market. All of this information provides insights vital to understanding an organization's current position and developing a strategic agenda for growth.

Chapter 5

Operational Considerations in Planning

Operational considerations in planning typically have centered around facilities, with boards focusing on whether to add, renovate, or relocate services and space. However, the current challenges facing health care entities affect virtually every aspect of an organization. Operational considerations are playing an increasingly important role in planning, and these considerations have broadened considerably beyond facilities issues. This chapter explores the operational considerations in strategic thinking and planning for health care organizations.

Comparative Performance

As described in chapter 1, health care payers are increasingly channeling or directing patients to provider organizations that offer the best "value" (for example, the best combination of price and quality). Because of this trend, it is imperative that a health care organization planning for its future should be able to assess its performance relative to other providers and incorporate the results of that assessment into its strategic thinking and planning. Although the board has a wide variety of factors upon which to base and compare its organization's performance, three key factors are (1) the cost and price of the services provided by the organization, (2) the quality of those services, and (3) the organization's efficiency in providing those services. In evaluating these three areas, the board should determine how its organization stacks up against other organizations in the market area, as opposed to determining how current organizational performance compares to its past performance over a specific period of time.

With respect to comparative cost performance, most health care organizations lack the data necessary to make accurate comparisons regarding their own cost position, not to mention the comparative data to determine the cost position of other area providers. In fact, many insurers and managed care organizations (and, increasingly, many employers) have more data on the costs and prices of area providers than do the providers themselves. Health care organizations have focused their attention on managing departmental costs rather than focusing on the cost per patient or per episode of treatment. Health care organizations should strive to determine their costs per patient and per episode of treatment and compare those costs to the costs of other organizations serving the community's health care needs.

The data sources available to health care organizations for the purpose of conducting cost comparisons vary according to each organization's location and the data collection capabilities of local and regional regulatory agencies, but more sources are becoming available every day. The board's role in conducting cost comparisons is to evaluate their organization's relative cost position, the changes in that cost position over time, and the corrective action plan devised by the organization's management.

Quality and outcomes measurement are becoming increasingly important to the health care environment of the 1990s. The measures used to determine quality and outcomes now extend beyond unsophisticated indicators such as the determination of mortality rates for the entire organization to the determination of service-specific (for example, for open-heart surgery) and physician-specific mortality rates. In addition, health care organizations are developing practice profiles of their professionals that provide those professionals with information regarding their use of resources, as well as comparisons to the practices of their peers.

To determine how its performance compares to the performance of other organizations serving the same community, a health care organization must define and assess performance indicators. The health care organization must determine what its new "customers," managed care organizations, want. Determining what managed care organizations use as quality indicators and incorporating those indicators into a health care organization's comparative performance analysis are critical to any organization's improvement process.

Medical Manpower and Human Resources

A significant percentage of a health care organization's costs relate to the organization's personnel, and its remaining costs are driven to a significant degree by the decisions of the organization's medical professionals. Therefore, the boards of health care organizations must carefully consider the current and anticipated availability of medical manpower and human resources.

With respect to medical manpower, board members need to assess the following issues and ask themselves many questions:

- *Age profile:* How many physicians will retire within the next 5 years? How many will retire within the next 10 years? What percentage of the organization's business do these professionals represent? This issue is important given the relative productivity of medical professionals at different points in their careers and their importance to and reliance on the health care organization.
- *Specialty mix:* What percentage of the organization's medical professionals are primary care physicians and what percentage are specialty physicians? As managed care continues to grow in importance in the health care field, the organization's physician mix will need to shift to at least 50 percent primary care physicians. Many managed care organizations seek a 60 percent primary care physician mix.
- *Location:* How accessible are the organization's medical professionals to the market? Where are their offices located? Access to population centers is very important, and the health care organization should discourage the tendency of many medical professionals to locate as near as possible to the organization. Locating offices close to the health care organization artificially restricts the patient draw to an area immediately surrounding the facility.
- *Practice mode:* Are the organization's medical professionals in solo or group practice? If they are in solo practice, can they be encouraged to form groups? Can existing groups be encouraged to form larger groups? Can the organization establish groups that physicians new to the area can join? Few medical professionals are interested in establishing solo practices or working in solo practices. (In recent surveys, fewer than 8 percent of recent medical school graduates indicated an interest in setting up solo practices.[1])
- *Activity levels:* How much volume does the medical professional generate for the organization? Activity-level indicators help measure a medical professional's commitment to the organization and what percentage of his or her patients are admitted to other health care organizations.
- *Managed care involvement:* How much managed care savvy does the medical professional possess? What percentage of his or her volume comes from managed care? Managed care represents a growing percentage of virtually every health care organization's volume, and an organization's future success will require a good working knowledge of the concepts and incentives of managed care. In addition, success in a managed care environment will require individuals and organizations to view managed care organizations as a customer rather than as an "enemy" to realize ultimate success. Individuals and organizations that are "managed care aware" will need to evolve into individuals and organizations that are "managed care aware" and "managed care friendly."

In addition to assessing the organization's internal medical manpower resources, the board should obtain an evaluation of the supply of and need for medical professionals in the market area served by the organization. This assessment of external medical manpower will enable the board to determine how area health care needs are being addressed and whether the organization will have access to the manpower resources necessary to implement the board's strategic plan. Additionally, this evaluation will help the board decide whether the organization will need to recruit additional medical professionals to the area.

As mentioned in chapter 1, *health care* is principally the activity of people caring for other people. Therefore, one of the major challenges facing the board of any health care organization is to ensure that the organization has the appropriate number and mix of people to provide care to the people who need care. This challenge will become more difficult in the future because, according to changing population demographics, the number of people in the age bracket that typically represents the majority of caregivers (that is, age 25 to 34) will decline.

The fact that health care organizations will have to compete for a smaller supply of caregivers has several implications for the areas of recruitment, retention, and reengineering. Specifically, health care organizations will likely find themselves engaged in aggressive recruitment campaigns, many of which will extend nationally (and perhaps even internationally) in an effort to find the right number and mix of professionals and skill sets. Because of strong competition for a limited supply of professionals, health care organizations will need to develop specific retention strategies. Among the lessons learned from recent personnel shortages is that health care organizations need to provide their employees and professionals with something more than a paycheck in order to avoid the prospect of fighting an escalating salary war. A major thrust in the effort to avoid such a salary war is examining the work performed by staff members and determining whether there are ways to do that work more efficiently and effectively. Reengineering a health care organization's work processes can substantially affect its human resource needs and work satisfaction levels.

The board should tap the knowledge base of current staff members when devising recruitment, retention, and reengineering strategies and processes. The need to "empower employees" may have become a cliché, but empowerment can produce strong results when executed correctly. Although involving an organization's staff members and professionals in recruiting, retention, and reengineering processes is difficult, this involvement can produce significant benefits, including higher satisfaction levels and greater productivity. Not only will tapping into the creativity and talent of staff members and professionals help the board and management find the right solutions to human resources challenges, but this involvement will also facilitate implementation of these solutions. These solutions are the ideas of staff members and professionals, and they have a sense of ownership in the solutions and a vested interest in making them work.

Physical Plant Resources

The location in which health care is rendered is shifting rapidly due to technological advances, new payment schemes, and regulatory changes. Many futurists predict that the majority of health care will eventually be delivered in the home. Nevertheless, most health care organizations have a substantial investment in facilities, and these facilities will continue to be important to the delivery of care, even if they are no longer the center of the health care delivery system.

During the strategic planning and thinking process, it is important for the board to evaluate the overall status of the organization's facilities, especially in terms of their accessibility to the patient population. Accessibility is increasingly important in an environment that is dominated by managed care (and reform) and that emphasizes convenience as a key attribute. As a result, not only must the board evaluate the accessibility of the organization's facilities relative to key patient populations, it also must evaluate accessibility relative to the enrollees of major managed care organizations. When evaluating accessibility, the board must consider features such as location, hours of operation, parking, safety, and signage and visibility.

The physical condition of facilities is also important to consider during the strategic planning and thinking process. Boards of health care organizations should objectively examine the condition of facilities to determine their functionality, expandability, and appearance. Additionally, boards should assess the potential obsolescence of facilities, especially in relation to changes in care modality (for example, increased outpatient volumes).

Health care is a healing art, and the healing process is affected by the type of setting in which care is delivered. Because more and more people are recognizing that "institutional" settings are not conducive to the healing process, boards of health care organizations should look for ways to humanize their facilities and make them more patient friendly. In addition to helping the healing process, a humane environment will make the facilities more attractive places for people to work.

Information Systems Resources

Integrated delivery systems are becoming more and more prominent in the health care field, and information is the "glue" that holds integrated delivery systems together. Despite this trend, most boards of health care organizations have paid little attention to information technology (IT) because of its inherent complexity and tremendous cost. As integrated delivery networks increasingly influence the health care field, there will be a growing need for board members to address IT issues directly during the strategic thinking and planning process.

Information technology will represent the lifeblood of the health care organization in the future. The board should determine where the organization's information system is in its life cycle (in relation to the system's estimated useful life) and begin planning for the upgrades and replacements necessary for the system to optimally function in an integrated delivery environment. Information technology upgrades and replacements can cost several million dollars. During the strategic thinking and planning process, the board should answer the following IT questions:

- Does IT assist in making informed strategic decisions?
- What percentage of the organization's operating budget is allocated to IT?
- What information does the board really need, and is the board receiving that information?

Many of the data provided to boards of health care organizations are less useful than they should be because the volume of data is overwhelming and the data are almost always organized around historical trends. More than anything else, boards need information regarding the current and future status of key indicators in order to monitor the performance of their organizations.

Summary

An understanding of how a health care organization operates and compares to other area providers, as well as its human resources, physical plant, and information system, is essential for strategic thinking and planning in today's health care environment. A clear sense of a health care organization's core competencies provides the board with a solid basis for testing and validating the potential benefits of implementing a given strategy.

Reference

1. Jolly, P., and Hudley, D. M., editors. *AAMC Data Book: Statistical Information Related to Medical Education.* Washington, DC: Association of American Medical Colleges, 1992.

Chapter 6

Financial Considerations in Planning

Financial considerations in planning have traditionally centered around capital expenditures such as facilities projects and major equipment purchases. Such considerations often occurred after the strategic plan was developed, in a process separate from that of strategic planning. Over the past 20-plus years, payment for capital expenses has shifted from covering the full cost of capital to covering only a portion. Payment for operating expenses has moved in the direction of fixed (versus actual) fees based on case-specific rates, episodes of care, or per plan enrollee methodologies. These changes in how health care providers receive payment for their services and fund capital investments make it imperative that financial considerations are (1) broadened beyond issues related to capital expenditures and (2) integrated into all aspects of the strategic planning process. This chapter explores the financial considerations in strategic thinking and planning for health care organizations. Because the changing health care environment has caused financial issues to assume tantamount importance for health care organizations, this chapter has been supplemented with a finance primer that includes a detailed explanation of how to read financial statements, important financial ratios, and debt capacity calculations and financing. (See the appendix.)

There are three major financial considerations in strategic thinking and planning:

1. The current and anticipated comparative financial performance of the organization
2. The strategic financial requirements of the organization
3. The interface between and integration of the strategic and financial activities of the organization

These financial considerations are discussed in the following sections.

Comparative Financial Performance

There are at least three ways that board members should comparatively assess their organization's financial performance:

1. Against the organization's historic financial trends
2. Against national credit averages (those with whom the organization will compete for capital)
3. Against a base-case scenario of future financial results if no strategic activities are undertaken (that is, if "business as usual" continues)

In order to complete each of the preceding assessments, it will be necessary to understand and calculate the key liquidity, profitability, and leverage ratios identified and explained in the finance primer. These ratios are used to review and evaluate an organization's financial performance.

Assessing an organization's financial trends provides a view of the organization's overall financial condition. Comparing the organization's financial performance to national averages provides an indicator of what the organization's credit rating would be if it attempted to raise money in the debt markets on the merits of its current performance.[1]

The development of a base-case scenario provides a picture of the organization's future financial condition absent the execution of new or different strategies (that is, no change in services, operations, or market focus). In completing a base-case scenario, several questions should be asked with respect to the external environment:

• How might area employers, including governments, alter the insurance coverage offered to their employees, and how might the payer mix (managed indemnity, HMO) be affected?
• In what ways are area payers likely to change their health care management and payment methodologies in the future, and what will be the impact of these changes on revenue?
• What volume changes might occur as a result of changing demographics?

The completion of a base-case scenario often functions as a catalyst for change because its resulting projections of financial performance are often far worse than performance that is currently being experienced. The board should compare the organization's financial position in the base-case scenario to a projection of the organization's future financial position under the strategic initiatives contained in the strategic plan. This comparison will help the board assess the impact of the plan on the organization's financial position and should provide additional information for the board to use in assessing the plan's value.

In addition to forecasting the results of the base case and making comparisons to financial trends and national averages, health care organizations should identify the changes that will be necessary to close the gap between present performance and forecasted and/or comparative performance. The following questions will help identify these changes:

- How much and what type of volume will be required to offset expected changes in payer mix?
- How will expenses need to be reduced to offset expected changes in payment methods?
- How can liquidity ratios be improved in the short term to enhance creditworthiness?

Strategic Financial Requirements

An organization's strategic financial requirements include both annual financial requirements and long-term capital requirements. Annual financial requirements include the following:

- Annual capital expenditures to meet operating needs
- Changes in working capital
- Actual principal payments
- Incremental expansion of *debt capacity* (the capacity to incur additional debt to be market responsive and resilient to change)
- Increases in cash on the balance sheet to respond to change and to preserve creditworthiness[2]

Long-term capital requirements relate to capital expenditures and are determined by answering the following questions:

- What are the organization's strategic capital requirements?
- How much cash should be available?
- How much debt can be afforded?
- If there is a capital shortfall, how large is it and what profitability targets or operating changes are necessary to resolve it?
- From where will needed capital originate?[3]

Sensitivity analyses can be performed to assess the financial impact of changes to operations (for example, staffing levels), service mix (for example, outpatient versus inpatient service), or to any of the external variables mentioned earlier (that is, utilization, payer mix, and/or payment methods). The purpose of sensitivity analysis is not to try to anticipate and quantify each and every variable but to identify and understand the impact of key variables on the organization's financial position.

Often there is a tendency to "wait until after the strategic plan is finished" to develop the organization's financial requirements. However, waiting can be problematic for several reasons. First, a weak comparative financial position may indicate a need to concentrate on existing operations before undertaking expansion or diversification. Second, the qualification of financial requirements may point out a severe shortfall between capital requirements and available debt capacity and cash, and such a shortfall may indicate the need to rethink the strategies behind proposed expenditures or the strategic need to "partner" with another entity. Finally, developing financial requirements after the planning stage detracts from the strategies and plans developed by indicating that what will be done is what can be afforded, as opposed to indicating that the organization will figure out how to afford what needs to be done.

The Interface between an Organization's Strategic and Financial Activities

A health care organization's strategic thinking and planning process will require financial input, analyses, and projections. Care must be taken to prepare the financial information in terms of broad parameters so that the strategic planning process and its related creativity are not bogged down with too many number. At the same time, the information must provide meaningful strategic input. Such care will necessitate a close working relationship between the organization's planning and finance staff as well as involvement from finance staff throughout the strategic planning process.

The capital and operating budget processes will also require interface. Board members must ensure that planning outcomes (that is, strategies and initiatives) are incorporated into the organization's routine financial functions. Both capital and operating budgets should support the direction set by the strategic plan. Indeed, these budget processes will be made easier if a strategic plan is in place.

Finally, the board should annually assess the resources appropriated to strategic initiatives against those used to enhance already-existing operations. This assessment should include the following questions:

- How much has the organization invested in growth as a percentage of capital?
- What is the value to be added from these investments (through analysis of return on investment)?
- Is the specific approach taken to develop a strategic initiative the best means to do so (that is, through an analysis of alternative approaches, including a net present value analysis of alternatives)?

Summary

Considering comparative financial performance and strategic financial requirements and interfacing strategic and financial activities are essential for strategic thinking and planning in health care organizations. Understanding financial indicators is one of the most important keys to developing appropriate strategies for the future.

References

1. Kaufman, K., and Hall, M. *The Financially Competitive Healthcare Organization*. Chicago: Probus, 1994, p. 32.

2. Kaufman and Hall, pp. 17–18.

3. Kaufman and Hall, p. 21.

Organizational Considerations in Planning

Although it is not the most obvious consideration in strategic planning and implementation, the organization itself—its structure, functions, and relationships—should not be overlooked. Analysis of an organization reveals the organization's values. Specifically, the key aspects of an organization that require consideration during the planning process are its management structure, governance, medical staff relationships, and external relationships.

Management Structure

The operating structure of a health care organization reflects what its management considers to be important. For example, a hospital structure that includes off-site ambulatory care and home health care as "departments" may indicate that the hospital considers outpatient care to be in support of or subservient to inpatient care. Separate operational structures for off-site ambulatory care and home health would accord more seriousness and/or a greater business purpose to these areas. In assessing an organization's management and operating structures and the impact of those structures on planning strategies, the following qualities should be considered:

- The duplication of functions and opportunities to enhance synergy through the combination of similar areas, whether they are staff or line functions (for example, multiple departments performing similar functions, poorly utilized areas that could be consolidated, and so forth)
- The relationships among the key divisions, lines of business, and revenue generators (Is the structure reflective of the key product lines and revenue generators?)

- The general focus across various functions and across the continuum of care (evaluating horizontal versus vertical communication and coordination, regardless of division or setting, to address patient care needs)

Governance

A health care organization's governance structure, the structure's participants, and the areas of control within that structure all create a statement of what is important to the organization strategically. The following governance-related questions should be asked during the strategic planning process:

- What is the size of the board and the tenure of its members, and how do those qualities relate to the board's manageability and activity? Are decisions that consider various points of view made in a timely fashion? Is there substantial "new blood" on the board to challenge the status quo?
- How accurately do board members represent and reflect the organization's community in terms of the community's geography, socioeconomic characteristics, businesses, payer groups, and so forth? Are ethnic and racial groups, large and small employers, and health plans represented?
- What is the nature of the board's spending authority and approval processes? Is the board appropriately focused at a high level, leaving management to administer details and oversee smaller items?
- What is the governance structure's strategic planning involvement, and in what other direction-setting activities does the governance structure participate? Is the board performing the planning functions outlined in chapter 2?

The Joint Commission on Accreditation of Healthcare Organizations and other organizations may mandate specific requirements with respect to governance and strategic planning, and these requirements should also be considered.

Medical Staff Relationships

The types of relationships among hospitals and members of their medical staffs are increasing rapidly. Although the ways that physicians integrate with health care organizations vary according to different structures and situations, at least four areas require relationships among medical staff members and the health care organization in order to accomplish strategic initiatives:

1. *Program development:* Determining how the organization and medical staff should work together to understand and meet community needs; developing the needs assessment and program planning process; and identifying the medical staff's role in the process
2. *Resource development:* Identifying needed medical manpower resources, developing recruitment plans, and devising strategies for the retention of existing resources
3. *Channel development:* Building an ongoing relationship with payers, employers, and other market channels
4. *Clinical care development:* Managing the delivery of medical care, which includes protocol development, utilization management, quality and outcomes measurement, and the creation of relevant credentialing standards

External Relationships

A final organizational consideration is how the health care organization interacts with external entities, especially in regard to community citizenship and the development of capabilities that enhance the organization's caliber and range of services. The board should consider the organization's role in the following external activities:

- *Community health:* Screenings, preventive services, and speakers
- *Community development:* Activities to help ensure the community's economic viability (for example, neighborhood development and professional training of local residents)
- *Education and training:* Assistance to students, interns, residents, and fellows
- *Service outreach:* Services for special population groups in conjunction with other health services (for example, emergency medical services and nursing homes)

Summary

Organizational considerations in planning should include management structure, governance, medical staff relationships, and external relationships. These areas reflect the organization's values and will greatly affect the chances for successful implementation of strategic plans.

Chapter 8

Strategic Assessment

Crafting a strategy in response to the realities of today's rapidly changing health care marketplace is a complex and critically important undertaking. Experience has shown that the most successful strategic plans focus simultaneously on the following three factors:

1. *Content:* Information regarding the market, other market-area providers, and customers
2. *Process:* Participation and acceptance by both internal and external constituencies
3. *Direction setting:* Desired future position, service complement and configuration, and structure

This chapter describes the strategic assessment component of the planning process—described as *content* in the preceding list. However, because this book is intended to provide an overview of the planning process rather than a detailed description of how to perform planning, this chapter focuses less on the "what" and "how" of the strategic assessment and more on the emphasis and orientation of the strategic assessment.

Purpose of the Strategic Assessment

The purpose of the strategic assessment is to provide planning participants with the following information:

- A common understanding of current and anticipated market dynamics
- An objective evaluation of the organization's core competencies
- A clear picture of where the organization stands relative to the market as it looks today and as it may look *in the future*

This assessment helps planners identify the critical strategic issues facing the organization and sets the stage for the development of a strategic vision to guide the organization's future.

In assessing its strategic position, a health care organization needs to consider quantitative input (factual data) and qualitative input (perceptions and opinions). Incorporating both types of input into the assessment process is critical because neither the quantitative nor the qualitative data provide a complete picture of market dynamics or the organization's capabilities. Combining the qualitative information with the quantitative data balances the strategic assessment. Planning processes that are overly reliant on qualitative input can lapse into the "group-grope syndrome," which often leads to a pooling of common myths. Processes that stick to "nothing but the facts" often miss the subtleties and nuances behind the statistics.

Another key element of the strategic assessment is the consideration of the implications and potential impact of major health care trends, as well as local trends, on the organization. Strategic assessment data and analyses are relevant only to the extent that planners continually ask what resultant trends mean to the organization and what influence the trends will have on the future environment of the organization.

Furthermore, because it is impossible to precisely predict the future, the strategic assessment should explore various what-ifs and consider their potential impact on the organization's strategy. Considering alternative future scenarios and determining what the organization would have to do differently in such environments can help prepare the organization for the uncertainties that lie ahead and discourage complacency.

Quantitative Input

Because of the increasing pace of change and the corresponding decline in stability in the health care field, assessing a health care organization's strategic position has become easier and more difficult at the same time. In less volatile times, health care data were less complete, more difficult to obtain, and less likely to become obsolete quickly. Most health care organizations had plenty of time to assess whatever data they could obtain regarding the market and their own internal situations.

During the 1980s, the explosion in and proliferation of personal computer technology, combined with the increased availability of data, caused many planning efforts to drown in a sea of data. In addition, partly owing to the relative stability of the health care field and the increased use of spreadsheets and projection software, strategic assessments often focused primarily, if not exclusively, on historical data. Organizations struggled to wade through pounds of paper in order to ponder the past.

Today, health care organizations have access to a great deal of data, most of which is historical, but have little time to assess that data and make increasingly important decisions regarding their futures. Extensive data tend to complicate, rather than simplify, decision making, because making and implementing decisions in a fast-paced, rapidly changing environment requires superior information and analysis, not merely more data. Additionally, the dramatic changes and shifts in the health care environment and most local markets prevent the extrapolation of historical trends in a neat linear-regression fashion. Planning in the chaotic world of health care requires more than exhaustive analysis of historical data: health care planning requires a focus on the current market and where it is going. Strategic assessments should emphasize the future state of the market as much as (if not more than) they emphasize the past and current state of the market.

Chapters 4 through 7 discussed the key areas and factors that must be considered in developing a strategic plan. Much of the information related to these key factors is quantitative and reflects the competitive dynamics in the market served by the organization and the organization's service delivery, operational, and financial capabilities. Many organizations structure their strategic assessments along these lines, with separate analyses related to external and internal factors.

In assessing the quantitative data relevant to the strategic assessment, health care organizations should start at the general, or macro, level and work down to the specific, or micro, level. For example, in examining external factors, organizations should first analyze industrywide and national trends and then move on to state, regional, and local issues and implications. When considering internal factors, assessments should begin at the institutional level and end up at the program-specific level.

As noted previously, the assessment of quantitative trends should determine the direction of trends and predict their implications for and impact on the organization. Data for the external components of the strategic assessment are generally available from a variety of sources, including the federal government, state agencies and organizations, professional associations and societies, trade associations, and private companies and firms. Information regarding an organization's services, human resources, and operational and financial performance is typically available from the organization's own information systems. However, data for the internal components of the strategic assessment are often maintained by separate departments, sometimes on different computer systems, and should be checked for internal consistency as well as for consistency with data reported by outside organizations and agencies.

In dealing with the quantitative data elements of the strategic assessment, health care organizations will need to strike a balance between the "need for speed" required in today's rapidly changing health care environment and the "paralysis of analysis" associated with the quest for complete and accurate data. The purpose of strategic planning is to make decisions based on information derived from data, not merely to develop a comprehensive, absolutely accurate database. Although data should be as accurate and complete as possible, the market will not wait while organizations attempt to gather every bit of data and resolve all of their inconsistencies and discrepancies. Health care organizations should collect all *available* quantitative data elements, identify and acknowledge their shortcomings, and determine the potential implications of the trends derived from the data.

Qualitative Input

In addition to focusing the quantitative portion of the strategic assessment on future trends, another major aspect of the strategic assessment is the inclusion of qualitative information regarding the marketplace and the organization. Because health care organizations are people organizations, it is critical to proactively seek input from the organization's key constituency groups during this phase of strategic assessment.

Obtaining input from key constituency groups can be accomplished in a variety of ways, depending on the size of the constituency groups and the fiscal constraints of the organization. Table 8-1 illustrates some of the techniques typically used to obtain the insights, perceptions, and suggestions of an organization's constituency groups. Each of the research techniques listed in table 8-1 can be appropriate in a given situation, but a health care organization should seek the advice of an individual or firm experienced in conducting primary research prior to using a particular research technique.

The opinions and perceptions of constituency groups provide valuable insights that complement the quantitative findings regarding market dynamics and the organization's core competencies. In some planning processes, health care organizations use qualitative input to probe issues that result from the quantitative data gathered. (For example: Why has our market position eroded? Why has our payer mix changed?) In other processes, quantitative data are used to determine whether common perceptions are in fact true. (For example: Our organization is the most inexpensive provider. Our organization is the provider most preferred by the community.)

The perceptions and opinions of a health care organization's constituency groups should be gathered on a regular basis (for example, annually or semiannually). This regular assessment of perceptions and opinions will allow the organization to create benchmarks for itself with regard to key qualitative factors and track its progress in addressing these factors over time.

Table 8-1. Potential Research Techniques

Constituency Group	Research Technique				
	Personal Interview	Telephone Interview	Telephone Survey	Mail Survey	Focus Group
Board	X	X			
Management	X				
Medical staff	X		X	X	X
Department directors				X	X
Employees				X	X
Community leaders	X				
Consumers			X		X
Employers	X	X		X	
Insurers	X	X			

Financial Forecasting

The long-standing tendency of health care organizations to segregate financial planning from strategic planning is inappropriate and shortsighted. Strategy and finance are intrinsically linked and interdependent. A brilliant but unfunded strategy is as ineffective in ensuring an organization's future as an organization with funding but no sense of how to use that funding. The health care organization that fully integrates its strategic and financial planning functions will ensure that its strategies are contributing to the financial success of the organization and that its financial resources are being allocated to activities supportive of the organization's strategic direction. A strategic assessment should include the following financial components:

- A baseline projection of the organization's financial position under a status quo or momentum scenario. (A *momentum scenario* is a projection in which an organization's existing financial situation and existing market trends are rolled forward for comparative purposes.) This analysis will help assess the impact of current trends and practices on the organization and will provide a point of comparison.
- An estimation of the organization's capacity to fund new initiatives, often referred to as *debt capacity*.
- A determination of the organization's cost position, leverage, and efficiency relative to other market area providers.

As with the analysis of quantitative data, these financial analyses should emphasize the organization's future financial position and capabilities. Financial forecasting will provide the organization with additional quantitative data relative to its market position and capabilities and will help ensure that the strategies developed by the organization will be realistic and affordable.

Scenario Building

Even the most exhaustive analysis of mounds of quantitative and qualitative data, combined with the collective insights and wisdom of board members, physicians, managers, professional planners, and consultants, cannot accurately predict future trends or divine *the* strategic direction of a health care organization in today's rapidly changing and unpredictable environment. A key element of focusing the strategic assessment on future issues involves asking the question: What if? Specifically, as part of the strategic assessment, planners should ask themselves what their organizations would do differently if the world in which they operate changed radically or if something were to create a world different than the one currently *anticipated*. This process of asking what if is called *scenario building*.

Scenario building is a relatively new technique based on the premise that even with all the information compiled and analyzed during the strategic assessment process, neither future market dynamics nor a health care organization's future performance can be predicted accurately. Yet quantitative and qualitative data do provide a sense of the range of potential futures facing the organization. Scenario building posits several plausible scenarios that incorporate key local, regional, and national trends. All of these scenarios (usually no more than six) are then assessed, not for how likely they are to become reality, but rather for what the organization would have to do to be successful assuming that a particular scenario actually occurred. Scenarios can be global (What would happen if the United States adopted a single-payer health system similar to Canada's system?) or local (What would happen if another market-area provider merged with the area's largest HMO?). During the scenario-building process, planning participants should focus on the following questions:

- What would the organization need to do differently if it were forced to operate in an environment different from its current environment or from the environment anticipated in the future?
- How would the structure of the organization need to change?
- Who would the organization's customers be, and what would those customers want?

- How and where would the organization serve its customers?
- Who would the organization's suppliers be? How would the organization work with those suppliers?
- What would the critical success factors be in each scenario?

The objective of scenario building is to prepare an organization to cope with an unpredictable future by examining various hypothetical future scenarios and exploring what the organization would do differently in those scenarios.

Critical Issues Identification

After compiling and analyzing the qualitative and quantitative input regarding the market and the organization's comparative strategic position, the challenge confronting board members and other planning participants is to distill their findings into a set of strategic critical issues. Although there are a number of methods to identify these critical issues (for example, brainstorming and the Delphi technique), planners should be sure to use the findings and major implications of the quantitative and qualitative data to highlight the issues that, if not addressed, could impair the organization's future growth and development. Typically, these issues number between 4 and 7 and should be kept to fewer than 10.

It is important to note that the strategic assessment is designed to identify—not resolve—critical planning issues. Once these issues have been identified, they form the core around which the organization will focus in the strategy-development portion of the planning process.

Summary

The output of the strategic assessment is a summary of the following findings:

- The potential future impact of major market trends on the organization
- The organization's strategic resources and core competency areas
- The needs and perceptions of key constituency groups
- The critical planning issues facing the organization as a result of changing market dynamics and organizational core competencies

The results of strategic assessment provide board members and other planning participants with a common understanding of the current and future market drivers and the competitive market position of the organization relative to the key drivers and other market-area providers. This common understanding of the issues will facilitate the development of a high-level statement of strategic direction.

Despite the improved availability of quantitative and qualitative data, board members who are involved in other industries, particularly service industries, may be somewhat surprised, dismayed, and even frustrated by the lack of comprehensive and timely information in the health care field. This information deficit is largely the result of the health care field's long-time underinvestment in information technology, particularly in comparison to other service industries. This lack of health care data is particularly obvious in areas that have exploded in size and importance during the past few years, including outpatient services, managed care participation, physician office activity, and cost information.

Although timely, accurate, and complete data in the areas critically important to today's health care field are often difficult to obtain, the absence of such data should not derail or delay the planning process. Board members and management teams must meet the challenge of making immediate decisions about the future without access to complete or timely information by collecting what relevant data elements they can in a timely manner, noting the limitations of such data, and pushing forward, looking for overall trends and identifying potential future changes in the trends. In addition, board members should recognize and address underinvestment in information technology as part of the strategic planning process.

Dealing with underinvestment in information technology will be expensive but essential. Board members should view dollars spent to enhance information technology as an investment in their organization's competitive capabilities rather than simply as an expense. Health care leaders would do well to learn from leading companies in other industries (for example, Wal-Mart®) that have used information technology to provide what customers want when and where the customers want it, at a lower cost than their competitors, because of—not in spite of—their investment in information technology.

Chapter 9

Strategy Development

After the assessment of the organization's strategic position, the next step in the health care strategic planning process is to establish a strategy to guide the organization's future development. Because the health care field is undergoing rapid and dramatic change, this component of the planning process must shift from the traditional focus on facility and program development to a focus on redefining the organization's core business and identifying new ways of operating. The challenge for the board and management is to craft a strategy that capitalizes on the changing market dynamics and the organization's capabilities (as defined in the strategic assessment) and to do so in a timely manner. This chapter discusses the board's role in identifying strategic alternatives for the organization, assessing those alternatives in light of strategic market trends and organizational core competencies, and crafting a vision for the organization.

Identifying and Assessing Strategic Alternatives

Health care organizations, like other businesses, cannot operate and compete successfully by attempting to be all things to all people. This maxim has never been more true than in the increasingly resource-constrained environment in which health care organizations find themselves today. Developing and maintaining a competitive advantage requires focus. One of the board's responsibilities in the planning process is to ensure that the organization is focused and that this focus is appropriate given market factors and the organization's internal resources. In order to fulfill this responsibility, the board needs to review the potential courses of action available to the organization and choose the most appropriate alternative on the basis of a structured and organized process.

As chapter 8 described, the strategic assessment portion of the planning process requires board members and other planners to distill data on external market factors and internal operational considerations into a series of issues confronting the organization. *Strategy development* is the process of deciding which issues are the most critical to the organization's future. The more specific process of developing *strategic alternatives* requires the organization to identify potential strategies it could follow to address each of the most critical issues.

Most health care organizations' strategic alternatives have typically centered around scope of service, level of technology, and geographic orientation, and most organizations have opted for pursuing a greater scope of service, higher levels of technology, and a broader geographic orientation. For example, some hospitals have chosen to become tertiary medical centers. Other hospitals have restructured their scopes of service to fit a highly focused market niche and have increased their technology levels and geographic orientations to support that restructuring. Today, health care organizations generally have more strategic issues with which to cope and hence more strategic alternatives. Scope of service, level of technology, and geographic orientation are still among the critical issues for health care organizations, but added to this list are often issues such as affiliation, risk assumption, and physician integration.

There are several ways to identify the strategic alternatives, ranging from informal discussion, to facilitated brainstorming, to more structured, analytical techniques. There is no one right way to identify strategic alternatives, but it is important to identify as wide a range of realistic alternatives as possible and avoid dismissing alternatives without giving each one appropriate consideration. In this regard, one of the board's roles in strategic thinking and planning for a health care organization is to ensure that the organization has identified all of the realistic strategic alternatives available.

Once the strategic alternatives have been identified, the board's responsibility is to review and assess the alternatives and reach a consensus regarding the organization's strategic direction based on its core competencies and market opportunities. Because these alternatives are actually a series of interrelated strategic issues, the evaluation and selection process encompasses a number of decisions regarding issues such as the following:

- Type of business definition
- Nature of geographic orientation (for example, markets served)
- Scope of services offered
- Level of affiliation with other organizations
- Degree of physician integration
- Level of risk assumption

As with the identification of alternatives, there is no single right way to assess strategic alternatives. How organizations approach this assessment should be a function of their organizational cultures. Some organizations utilize a process that establishes a series of criteria against which strategic alternatives can be evaluated. The following list provides examples of such criteria:

- Provides consistency with organizational mission
- Creates responsiveness to market needs and opportunities
- Leverages organizational strengths
- Addresses organizational weaknesses
- Addresses weaknesses in the range of services provided by all market-area providers
- Ensures political acceptability
- Maximizes financial risk–return potential

Some health care organizations add weights to these types of criteria and score each alternative using the weighted criteria. Other organizations prefer to use facilitated group processes to reach a consensus. Still other organizations are employing interactive computer polling technologies to determine the preferred strategic alternative. Regardless of the method used to evaluate and select strategic alternatives, the board must ensure that the alternatives evaluated are appropriate on the basis of the organization's strategic assessment and that the evaluation process is conducted objectively.

Crafting a Vision

Once its strategy is determined, an organization must craft a vision statement that builds on the critical strategic issues discussed and articulates how the organization needs to change to meet future challenges. The board's role in crafting a vision can vary from actively participating in the development of the vision to reviewing and revising a draft prepared by management or a planning committee. Whatever means are used to craft the vision statement, the board's responsibilities are to ensure that the vision is consistent with the organization's mission and that it is appropriate for the organization.

As noted in chapter 3, the vision statement of an organization differs from its mission. A *mission* defines the reason the organization exists and is usually broad and durable over time. An organization's *vision statement* is more directional and temporal and focuses on the organization's future. In other words, the vision statement is a high-level description of the desired future state of the organization. However, an organization's mission and vision statement need to be consistent with one another, and, in fact, the vision statement should help identify how the organization will accomplish its mission.

In addition to ensuring that the vision statement is consistent and appropriate, the board should ensure that the vision is based on the unique decisions made regarding the organization's previously identified critical issues. These decisions represent the foundation upon which the vision statement stands. It is important for board members to remember that the methodology used to evaluate a health care organization's vision statement cannot be imported from an organization in another market area, even when both organizations' circumstances seem very similar. Every market has unique drivers and dynamics, and attempting to craft a vision statement based on vision statements of organizations in other market areas almost invariably creates problems, not the least of which are lost time, energy, and credibility. As Michael Porter wrote in his book *Competitive Strategy: Techniques for Analyzing Industries and Competitors,* "The best strategy for a given firm is ultimately a unique construction reflecting its particular circumstances."[1]

Vision statements can take many forms, but whatever their form, they require three important qualities:

1. *A futuristic orientation:* The vision statement should focus on the future and describe what the organization "wants to be when it grows up." Although organizational mission statements tend to focus on internal issues because they at least partially emphasize historical circumstances, well-crafted vision statements are more externally focused because they emphasize the future. Most people are excited by and optimistic about the future, and a futuristic orientation can help inspire and motivate a health care organization's workforce. Most people realize that, even though they cannot change an organization's past, they can help shape its destiny.
2. *Comprehensibility:* To be effective, a health care organization's vision statement must be meaningful to everyone in the organization, no matter what level they occupy in the organization's structure. A vision statement that is comprehensible only to the senior-level managers and board members who wrote it will not help an organization succeed in the highly competitive health care environment of the future. This is because much of the implementation of the vision will ultimately take place in the proverbial trenches of the organization. If the people who are responsible for implementing the vision do not understand it or believe it is necessary, then it is doubtful that the vision can be successfully implemented.
3. *Conciseness:* Vision statements need not be lengthy; in fact, shorter is better. The length of the vision statement is not nearly as important as its ability to be easily understood and to help each person in the orga-

nization put his or her contribution to the vision into perspective. The importance of conciseness and its role in putting a vision into perspective is perhaps best exemplified by the story of the traveler who happened across three masons hard at work. When queried as to what they were doing, the first mason replied, "Laying bricks." The second mason responded, "Building a wall." The third mason paused and then said, "I'm building a cathedral." To be successful, health care organizations need people who are building cathedrals, not merely laying bricks or building walls.

In addition to ensuring that the vision statement of their organization is future oriented, comprehensible, and concise, board members should ensure that the vision statement is meaningful to their particular organization. Developing a vision statement that is unique and applicable to only one organization is a difficult and perhaps unnecessary challenge. Although it is essential that the vision be developed by and for the organization, it is unlikely that the statement will be so specific that it could not be applied to other organizations. The important consideration for board members is not whether the vision statement applies only to their organization, but whether the vision statement makes sense for their organization.

Formulating Strategies

A vision statement must be translated into specific goals, objectives, and strategies if it is to achieve results and be seen as anything more than a statement. These goals, objectives, and strategies should be derived directly from the vision and should relate to the critical issues (often referred to as *focal areas*) identified earlier. (Typically, there are at least four and at most eight critical issues.)

Goals are usually general and take the form of an action (to-do) statement. Each focal area is supported by at least one goal and sometimes by several goals, although experience has shown that limiting the number of goals per focal area, as well as limiting the number of goals overall, is important in developing a plan that has a realistic chance of implementation. Each focal area goal is in turn supported by one or more measurable and time-based objectives specific to that goal. Finally, each of the objectives is supported by one or more strategies. These strategies articulate specifically how the individual objective will be achieved, which in turn indicates how the overall goal will be met.

The board's role in the planning process undergoes a subtle but important shift during the development of goals, objectives, and strategies. Specifically, although the board usually works with management in establishing goals for the focal areas, the board's role in developing objectives and strategies becomes one of oversight and review as opposed to actual formulation. The board sometimes participates in the establishment of objectives and strategies, but the board's main responsibility at this point in the planning process is to provide overall direction to the objective and strategy development process and to review the results of the process to ensure that the entire effort is integrated and coordinated.

There are numerous techniques for establishing objectives and developing strategies, including brainstorming. Another technique is to designate an action team made of individuals within the organization that have experience and knowledge in a particular area. These individuals are charged with identifying appropriate objectives and strategies supportive of the vision and goals established by the board.

The board's review function at this stage of the planning process includes three activities:

1. Reviewing each goal to ensure that it is directly tied to and supportive of the organization's vision
2. Reviewing each objective to ensure that it is reasonable and related to a specific goal
3. Reviewing each strategy to ensure that it is derived from and will help achieve an objective

This review sequence will ensure that every strategy ultimately refers back to the organization's vision.

Part of the board's role is to help its organization focus on the strategies, objectives, and goals that are critical to the organization's future. If a strategy cannot be directly traced back to an organization's vision through its objectives and goals, then the board should strongly question whether the strategy belongs in the plan.

Having established the overall direction of the organization by crafting the organization's vision and helping to establish related goals, objectives, and strategies, the board should be in a position to address questions such as the following:

- Given the organizational and operational strengths and limitations of the organization, as well as the market opportunities and challenges, what short-term (one to two years), intermediate (three to five years), and long-term (more than five years) options exist for ensuring the organization's future success?
- In light of expected changes in the local and regional marketplace, as well as in the national health care environment, what is the most appropriate vision for the organization?
- What type(s) of affiliation and/or strategic alliance, if any, should the

organization develop in order to maintain and further develop its position in the marketplace?

- What should the organization's stance toward and role in managed care be?
- What types of risk sharing should the organization undertake, and what levels of risk should it assume?
- What delivery system integration model(s) is appropriate for the organization given its capabilities and the market dynamics?
- What scope of services should the organization offer? To which market segments should those services be offered?

Testing Strategic Impact

Before board members can give final approval to their organization's vision, goals, objectives, and strategies, all of which have been formulated on the basis of what is achievable given marketplace realities and the organization's core competencies, those four planning components should be assessed to determine the potential impact they will have on the organization should they be successfully implemented. This assessment should compare the baseline projection developed in the strategic assessment (see chapter 8) with a "future-state" projection that incorporates the impact of the formulated strategies.

Future-state projections should incorporate estimates of the expenses (including major equipment, facilities, and personnel) and incremental revenues associated with the supporting strategies. These projections, which can be done on a strategy-specific basis and/or on an enterprisewide level, should be developed in conjunction with the organization's financial personnel and integrated with the organization's budgeting process. When a health care organization integrates its budgeting process with its planning process, the organization helps ensure that its strategic plan is achievable and that the related budgets are strategic. Although this integration may be difficult to achieve initially because of some health care organizations' autonomous departmental structures, the budgetary process ultimately should be driven by the strategic plan so that the organization is budgeting as the result of a plan and not planning as the result of a budget.

Regardless of whether a health care organization conducts its impact assessment on a strategy-specific basis or on an enterprisewide level, it is important that the assessment extend at least three (and preferably five) years into the future. This extended outlook is necessary to ensure a fair comparison between the baseline and future state projections because new strategic initiatives often require two to three years to reach break-even status. Furthermore, some of the plan's strategic initiatives are not even scheduled for implementation during the first year. Therefore, it is sometimes impossible to know the full impact of the initiatives until several years have passed.

Board members should also recognize that while they assess the impact of different plans on their organization, it may seem that their organization's financial situation can be made to appear quite positive in the near term by conserving capital and deferring appropriate investments. However, postponing appropriate strategic action to save money in the short term is ultimately counterproductive because every organization must make investments over time in order to remain viable and renew itself. Thus, although deferring investment may seem to bolster an organization's financial performance, its board members would do well to remember a venerable maxim: "It takes money to make money."

Another consideration for board members to keep in mind when assessing the organizational impact of different strategies is that not all strategies will be or are intended to be self-supporting. In fact, some strategies may be recommended in order to fulfill nonfinancial needs (for example, responding to identified community needs, social justice issues, and so forth). The board must assess each strategy's impact on the basis of what the strategy is intended to accomplish.

Finally, after the board exercises its strategy-assessment role and responsibility by reviewing the key assumptions used in the baseline and future-state projections for reasonableness and completeness and discussing the results of the impact assessment, the board must approve or modify the strategies. The board should recognize that modifying strategies at this point of the strategy-development process does not mean that the plan is intrinsically poorly developed. Rather, modifying the strategies before they have been implemented and before resources have been expended is highly preferable to trying to modify the plan after resources have been spent. Good planning processes always anticipate that some modifications will occur at this point as a result of the strategic impact analysis.

Summary

Strategy development represents one of the most challenging aspects of the board's role in the planning process. Developing strategy requires the board's active participation, but much of the board's responsibility during this phase is to work with management to craft an overall vision and a set of general goals and to review and revise (rather than develop by themselves) specific objectives and strategies designed to achieve the vision and goals. The board must delicately balance its role of establishing policy and setting direction with management's role of implementing that policy and direction. As the health care field becomes more volatile, the direction-setting function will take on an increasingly important role, as will the function of monitoring implementation.

Reference

1. Porter, M. E. *Competitive Strategy: Techniques for Analyzing Industries and Competitors*. New York City: The Free Press, 1980, p. 34.

Chapter 10

The Implementation Plan

When strategic plans fail, they usually do not fail because of inadequate analysis or inherent unsoundness. Strategic plans fail because they lack an implementation plan that translates the goals, objectives, and strategies of the health care organization into detailed and practical specifications that address the following questions:

- What tasks need to be accomplished?
- Over what period of time should the tasks be accomplished?
- Who should be responsible for ensuring that the tasks are accomplished?
- What resources are required to accomplish the tasks?

This chapter provides an overview of the implementation component of the strategic planning process. Because the development and execution of an implementation plan are managerial responsibilities, this chapter does not detail those subjects. Instead, this chapter describes the components of a well-designed implementation plan and discusses the board's role and responsibility in reviewing, approving, and monitoring the plan.

Components of the Implementation Plan

An organization's goals and objectives are supported by specific strategies, as discussed in chapter 9. These strategies must, in turn, be supported by an implementation plan that accomplishes the following:

- Identifies the tasks associated with each strategy
- Establishes a timetable for accomplishing each task
- Delineates the capital, facility, and organizational resources, as well as the human resources, necessary to implement the strategies
- Assigns responsibilities for strategy implementation

The implementation plan becomes the organization's agenda for change and provides the task-level direction necessary for the organization to grow into its envisioned "future state."

Although the management of the organization is usually charged with developing and executing the implementation plan, the board plays a critical role in reviewing, approving, and monitoring the plan. Specifically, the board has four key responsibilities:

1. The board should ensure that the implementation plan is consistent with and supportive of the organization's strategic direction. As part of this internal consistency check, the board should make sure that implementation tasks and timetables do not conflict with one another and that responsibilities are assigned in an appropriate and balanced manner.
2. The board should review the plan to determine whether the organization's critical issues are being adequately addressed and whether the organization's financial and human capital are being appropriately allocated.
3. The board should assess the implementation plan for realism. Many organizations' strategic plans try to accomplish too much, and as a result the plans actually accomplish very little because the organizations' resources are spread too thin. In addition, there is a natural tendency for organizations to schedule too many things too early in the implementation period. This leads to disenchantment with the plan and discouragement on the part of members of the organization because goals and objectives are not being accomplished. The board must keep the organization focused during the implementation phase of the strategic planning process.
4. The board should monitor the organization's progress in meeting its goals, objectives, and timetables. This responsibility is discussed further later in this chapter.

The Plan's Relationship to Other Planning and Management Functions

An implementation plan helps identify the resources a health care organization needs to be successful and is critical to the development of effective operating, capital, and cash flow budgets. In addition, an implementation plan helps ensure the development of relevant capital, facility, human resource, and information technology plans. Typically, most plans and management functions in health care organizations have been performed as discrete processes, with limited integration among plans or with the strategic planning process. Although the less chaotic health care market of the past allowed this separation of functions and plans, the current and future health care environment demands that these functions and plans be viewed and developed as highly interrelated components. In fact, only when all of its functions and plans are integrated will an organization be able to marshal its resources in a coordinated and effective manner.

Capital budgets and plans should reflect an organization's strategic direction by allocating resources to the strategic initiatives developed to help the organization achieve its goals and objectives. As capital becomes increasingly scarce and expensive, board members must ensure that their organization's capital is being allocated to those activities and initiatives that are directly tied to the organization's goals and objectives and thus help to achieve the organization's vision.

Similarly, a health care organization's facilities planning should be performed as a function of, rather than independently from, the strategic plan. The organization should first determine which functions it will perform and then develop the facilities in which to perform those functions. Health care boards should always remember the architectural maxim that form (facilities) follows function (strategy).

In terms of human resources, the strategic plan should help the health care organization identify the resources and skills needed to accomplish various tasks called for in the plan. This inventory of required resources and skills in turn provides valuable information for the organization's human resources plan, including data on recruitment priorities and needed training programs. Furthermore, as the organization develops a new vision, new goals, and new objectives, the organization's performance measurement and reward system must be aligned with the new vision, goals, and objectives.

Most health care organizations will have to make significant near-term investments in information technology in order to compete and thrive in an increasingly data-intense health care environment. The importance of information technology requires each health care organization to develop an information technology plan that is driven by the organization's strategic direction and that supports the organization's vision, goals, and objectives.

The board's role in the integration of the previously described management and planning functions is to ensure that true integration exists and that the plans are consistent with, supportive of, and directly linked to the organization's strategic plan. When evaluating whether and how planning and management functions relate to the strategic plan, the board should ask questions such as the following:

- How does this planning and/or management function relate to the organization as a whole, and how does the function help the organization achieve its strategic vision?

• What strategic goal(s) and/or objective(s) does this function support?

Some organizations even require that when a department or other organizational unit requests approval for a major capital, facility, human resources, or information technology initiative, the specific strategic goal or objective that the initiative supports must be identified. Additionally, the department or other organizational unit must describe how the initiative requested will help support that goal or objective.

Monitoring and Evaluating the Implementation Plan

To help the board monitor the implementation of the strategic plan, management (which is responsible for plan development and implementation) should provide the board with status reports regarding progress and any variances between the implementation plan and actual results. These status reports should be provided at least annually, but quarterly reports would be preferable. In addition to explaining the accomplishments and results of the implementation plan, the status reports should detail corrective plans of action for variances.

After monitoring the implementation plan for a period of time (for example, a quarter), the organization should extend the time horizon covered by the plan by the same period of time (for example, another quarter). The process of continual evaluation and the establishment of new evaluation time periods enables the organization to adjust the implementation plan in response to changing circumstances, which in turn prevents the plan from becoming obsolete. Furthermore, because the implementation plan's objectives are time based and measurable, the board can and should consider management's progress in implementing the plan when evaluating management performance and setting management compensation.

Until recently, health care organizations routinely developed long-range implementation plans that encompassed as many as 10 years. In today's health care marketplace, the scope and pace of change largely precludes planning horizons that extend beyond three years. An implementation plan should focus on a three-year horizon, although some of its initiatives may take longer to come to fruition, particularly initiatives that require regulatory approval, represent significant capital outlays, or commence during the second or third year of the planning horizon. Therefore, even though most of the plan's strategies will be initiated within the first three years of the planning horizon, the actual timetable of the implementation plan will likely be from five to seven years. While monitoring and evaluating the implementation plan, the board should not forget to revisit the organization's key market assumptions and major strategies on an annual basis and review and revise the organization's vision, goals, and objectives every three years.

Continuous Planning and Implementation

Even though solid implementation plans help ensure the success of a health care organization's strategic plans, strategic plans supported by well-developed implementation plans may still fail if they ignore the organization's human factors and other organizational issues. These human factors and organizational issues are particularly critical in a health care organization, where a broad range of constituencies must "buy in to" the organization's mission and direction in order for strategic plan implementation to be successful. To effectively address these factors and issues, the board must consider three implementation and planning principles during strategic plan development.

First, the implementation plan has the best chance for success if the people ultimately responsible for implementation understand the plan, are committed to making it successful, and believe that the changes encompassed in the plan will benefit them. To create this mind-set, the planning process should involve individuals from all areas of the organization through the establishment of focus groups, task teams, and problem-solving groups. These individuals can offer their perspectives and insights to the board as the implementation plan is being developed and help guide the plan and shape it into something that is achievable. The implementation plan then becomes their plan. These individuals have ownership in the plan and a vested interest in the plan's success.

Second, implementation must begin during the planning process itself. Although the average time required to complete the planning process has decreased in recent years from over nine months to less than six, the health care marketplace is relentless and will not wait for any organization to develop its strategy. The marketplace will present health care organizations with challenges and opportunities on a daily basis, and organizations must be prepared to respond. In today's fast-paced health care environment, quick decision making will be a critical success factor. Board members will need to be able to make decisions quickly and often without complete information. In these situations, board members must rely on their own instincts as well as those of the management team. However, board members must recognize that these rapid-response decisions will not always be the right decisions, and they should be willing to reverse a decision if circumstances change or if assumptions are proved wrong. The key consideration for the board is that for time-sensitive issues or the proverbial no-brainers, it may be impossible or unnecessary to wait for the completion of the planning process. In addition, the ability to make timely decisions and quickly begin implementation will build confidence in the board among an organization's constituency groups.

Third, the strategic planning process never really ends. Although the actual time frame within which the formal planning process occurs is typically three to six months, health care organizations and their boards should recognize that planning is an ongoing, continuous process.

Summary

The implementation plan is a key element in the successful strategic plan. It translates a health care organization's vision, goals, objectives, and strategies into specific action steps and specifies which people are responsible for implementation, as well as time frames for implementation results. Without a well-thought-out implementation plan, many strategic plans fail. As Peter Drucker wrote in his book *Management: Tasks, Responsibilities, Practices:*

> The best plan is only a plan, that is, good intentions, unless it degenerates into work. The distinction that marks a plan capable of producing results is the commitment of key people to work on specific tasks. The test of a plan is whether management actually commits resources to action which will bring results in the future. Unless such commitment is made, there are only promises and hopes, but no plan.[1]

Above all, the board's role and responsibility during this phase of the planning process is to review and approve the implementation plan developed by management and monitor management's execution of the plan.

Reference

1. Drucker, P. F. *Management: Tasks, Responsibilities, Practices.* New York City: Harper & Row, 1974, p. 128.

Chapter 11

Conclusion

Growing costs, competition, and price constraints, as well as the call for health care reform, have combined to place today's hospitals in a position of considerable economic risk. Although it is the responsibility of senior managers to ensure that their health care organization is positioned competitively and achieving operational excellence, the board of directors shares with management the responsibilities of ensuring that a sound, disciplined, and ongoing planning process is in place; that the organization has a clearly defined strategic direction; and that goals, strategies, and action plans are developed. The board also has the responsibility to monitor the results of implementation activities and compare those results to the plan's objectives and timetables.

The quality and effectiveness of a strategic plan depend on the planning process employed, the caliber of the participants involved in the process, and the degree of strategic thinking that takes place during the process. Solid market, operational, financial, and organizational information and projections are required to effectively assess the health care organization's current position and craft successful strategies for the organization's future. These strategies, along with the development of a realistic, achievable implementation schedule, form the foundation of a health care organization's strategic planning function.

A strategic plan will not create change in and of itself. The plan must be executed, monitored, and evaluated if it is to result in change. Like a compass, the strategic plan provides direction—it is a tool for helping the organization navigate the waters of the future.

The strategic planning process described in this book is not unique to health care organizations. There are numerous books and journal articles on strategic planning and related subjects that apply to health care organizations as well as to other types of business organizations. A list of suggested reading and reference materials is provided in the following section of this book for the reader who wishes to explore strategic planning further.

Suggested Reading
and References

Books and Articles

Alkhafaji, A. F. *A Stakeholder Approach to Corporate Governance: Managing in a Dynamic Environment.* New York: Quorum, 1989.

American Hospital Association. *The Future of Hospital–Physician Relations: Implications for Hospital Governance.* Chicago: AHA, 1989.

American Hospital Association. *The Guide to Governance for Hospital Trustees.* Chicago: AHA, 1990.

American Hospital Association. *Hospitals and Physicians in the Year 2000.* Chicago: AHA, 1990.

American Quality Foundation and Ernst & Young. *International Quality Study, Health Care Industry Report.* Cleveland: American Quality Foundation and Ernst & Young, 1992.

Bader, B. S. *Five Keys to Building an Excellent Governing Board.* Rockville, MD: Bader and Associates, with the Hospital Trustee Association of Pennsylvania, 1991.

Bader, B. S. *Informing the Board about Medical Staff Credentialing and Development.* Rockville, MD: Bader and Associates, with the Hospital Trustee Association of Pennsylvania, 1991.

Bader, B. S. *Informing the Board about Quality.* Rockville, MD: Bader and Associates, with the Hospital Trustee Association of Pennsylvania, 1991.

Bader, B. S. *Planning Successful Board Retreats: A Guide for Board Members and CEOs.* Washington, DC: National Center for Nonprofit Boards, 1991.

Bauer, E. I., and Harger, P. S. Assessing community needs: a system's six-step approach yields tangible results. *Health Progress* 75(1):54–59, Jan.–Feb. 1994.

Binns, G. S. The relationship among quality, cost, and market share in hospitals. *Topics in Health Care Financing* 18(2):21–32, Dec. 1991.

Blair, J. D., and Fottler, M. D. *Challenges in Health Care Management.* San Francisco: Jossey-Bass, 1990.

Blair, J. D., Savage, G. T., and Whitehead, C. J. A strategic approach for negotiating with hospital stakeholders. *Health Care Management Review* 19:13–23, Dec. 1989.

Brown, J. B., Thomas, S. R., and others. *Health Capital Financing: Structuring Politics and Markets to Produce Community Health.* Ann Arbor, MI: Health Administration Press, 1988.

Burns, M., and Mauet, A. R. Patrolling the turbulent borderland: managerial strategies for a changing health care environment. *Health Care Management Review* 14(1):7–12, Dec. 1989.

Campbell, A. B. Strategic planning in health care: methods and applications. *Quality Management in Health Care* 1(4):12–23, Summer 1993.

Chait, R. P., Holland, T. P., and Taylor, B. E. *The Effective Board of Trustees.* New York City: Macmillan, 1991.

Cleverley, W. O., editor. *Handbook of Health Care Accounting and Finance.* 2nd ed. Gaithersburg, MD: Aspen, 1989.

Coile, R. C., Jr. *The New Governance: Strategies for an Era of Health Reform.* Ann Arbor, MI: Health Administration Press, 1994.

Coile, R. C., Jr. *The New Medicine: Reshaping Medical Practice and Health Care Management.* Rockville, MD: Aspen, 1990.

Conrad, D. A., and Dowling, W. L. Vertical integration in health services: theory and managerial implications. *Health Care Management Review* 15:9–22, Sept. 1990.

Corley, W. E. Total quality, strategic planning, and community benefit: are they compatible or contradictory? *Quality Letter for Healthcare Leaders* 5(7):21–24, Sept. 1993.

Duncan, W. J., Ginter, P. M., and Swayne, L. E. *Strategic Issues in Health Care Management.* Boston: PWS-KENT, 1992.

Duncan, W. J., Ginter, P. M., and Swayne, L. E. *Strategic Management of Health Care Facilities.* Boston: PWS-KENT, 1992.

Ernst & Young. *Audit Committees, Functioning in the 1990s.* Cleveland: Ernst & Young, 1992.

Fisher, A. B. Is long-range planning worth it? *Fortune,* Apr. 23, 1990, pp. 281–84.

Folger, J. C. Integration of strategic, financial plans vital to success. *Healthcare Financial Management* 43:23–32, Jan. 1989.

Fottler, M., and others. Assessing key stakeholders: who matters to hospitals and why? *Hospital & Health Services Administration* 34:535–46, Dec. 1989.

Gall, E. A. Strategies for merger success. *The Journal of Business Strategy* 12(2):26–29, Mar. 1991.

Ginter, P. M., Duncan, W. J., Richardson, W. D., and Swayne, L. E. Analyzing the health care environment: "you can't hit what you can't see." *Health Care Management Review* 16(4):35–48, Sept. 1991.

Glenesk, A. E. Six myths that can cloud strategic vision. *Healthcare Financial Management* 44(5):38–43, May 1990.

Goldsmith, J. A radical prescription for hospitals. *Harvard Business Review,* May 1989, pp. 104–11.

Griffith, J. R. *The Well-Managed Community Hospital.* 2nd ed. Ann Arbor, MI: Health Administration Press, 1992.

Gyenes, L. A. Build the foundation for a successful joint venture. *The Journal of Business Strategy* 12(6):27–32, Nov. 1991.

Hains, C. T. The fiduciary responsibilities of the hospital board of directors. *Journal of Healthcare Quality* 15(1):36–41, Jan.–Feb. 1993.

Hastings, M. R. *Cost Management Strategies for Smaller Hospitals.* Chicago: American Hospital Publishing, 1993.

Henderson, B. D. The origin of strategy. *Harvard Business Review* 67:139–43, Nov. 1989.

Hiam, A. Exposing four myths of strategic planning. *The Journal of Business Strategy* 11(5):23–28, Sept. 1990.

Hospital Research and Educational Trust. *The Changing Character of Hospital Governance.* Chicago: HRET, 1990.

Hospital Research and Educational Trust. *Trustees and the Integration of Community Health Care.* Chicago: HRET, 1993.

Houle, C. O. *Governing Boards.* San Francisco: Jossey-Bass, 1989.

Johnson, D. E. Strategic thinking about collaboration and integration. *Health Care Strategic Management* 11(3):2–3, Mar. 1993.

Kazemek, E. A., and Grauman, D. M. Teamwork approach to strategy keeps CEOs in tune with players. *Health Care Strategic Management* 10(2)16–17, Feb. 1992.

Kovner, A. R. The case of the unhealthy hospital. *Harvard Business Review,* Sept. 1991, pp. 12–25.

Lorange, P., and Roos, J. Why some strategic alliances succeed and others fail. *The Journal of Business Strategy* 12(1):25–30, Jan. 1991.

MacKelvie, C. F., and Mauro, M. H. *The Trustee's Guide to Board Duties, Liabilities, and Responsibilities.* Chicago: Probus, 1993.

McComb, J. P., Jr. *Governing Community Hospitals.* San Francisco: Jossey-Bass, 1992.

McManis, G. L. Putting your strategic plan into effect. *Modern Healthcare* 21(2):40, Jan. 14, 1991.

McManis, G. L., and Stewart, J. A. Hospital collaboration: benefits for hospitals and for their communities. *Healthcare Executive* 6(3):7–9, May 1991.

Making strategic choices. *Integrated Healthcare Report,* Jan. 1993, pp. 1–7.

Nyp, R. G., and Angermeier, I. Financial plan charts a hospital's course for success. *Healthcare Financial Management* 44(5):30–36, May 1990.

Orlikoff, J. E., and Totten, M. K. *The Board's Role in Quality Care: A Practical Guide for Hospital Trustees.* Chicago: American Hospital Publishing, 1991.

Philbin, P. W. From the ground up: planting the seeds of network development. *Hospitals & Health Networks* 67(11):46–52, June 5, 1993.

Pointer, D. D., and Ewell, C. M. *Really Governing.* Albany, NY: Delmar, 1994.

Pratt, J. R. Defining and enhancing the medical staff's role in strategic planning. *Trustee* 46(1):14–15, Jan. 1993.

Preslar, L. B., Jr. Collaboration can work—given the right commitment. *Health Care Strategic Management* 10(11):13–16, Nov. 1992.

Rindler, M. E. *The Challenge of Hospital Governance: How to Become an Exemplary Board.* Chicago: American Hospital Publishing, 1992.

Robert, M. The do's and don'ts of strategic alliances. *The Journal of Business Strategy* 13(2):50–53, Mar. 1992.

Rovin, S., and Ginsberg, L., editors. *Managing Hospitals.* San Francisco: Jossey-Bass, 1991.

Salmon, W. J. Crisis prevention: how to gear up your board. *Harvard Business Review* 71(1):68–75, Jan.–Feb 1993.

Sandy, W. Avoid the breakdowns between planning and implementation. *Journal of Business Strategy* 12:30–33, Sept. 1991.

Scavatto, M. Strategic planning: using a matrix to help set priorities. *Trustee* 44(11):8–9, 21, Nov. 1991.

Seidel, L. F., Seavey, J. W., and Lewis, R. J. A. *Strategic Management for Healthcare Organizations.* Owings Mills, MD: AUPHA, 1989.

Shortell, S. M., Gillies, R. R., Anderson, D. A., Mitchell, J. B., and Morgan, K. L. Creating organized delivery systems: the barriers and facilitators. *Hospital Health Service Administration* 38(4):447–66, Winter 1993.

Smith, H. L., Piland, N. F., and Funk, M. J. Strategic planning in rural health care organizations. *Health Care Management Review* 17(3):63–80, Summer 1992.

Solovy, A. T., editor. *Hospital Capital Formation: Strategies and Tactics for the 1990s.* Chicago: American Hospital Publishing, 1990.

Spenner, D., editor. *Working Together to Shape the Future: Environmental Assessment 93/94.* Chicago: American Hospital Association, 1993.

Spiegel, A. D., and Hyman, H. H. *Strategic Health Planning.* Norwood, NJ: Ablex, 1991.

Tregoe, B. B., and Tobia, P. M. Strategy versus planning: bridging the gap. *The Journal of Business Strategy* 12(6):14–19, Nov. 1991.

Umbdenstock, R. J. *So You're on the Hospital Board!* 4th ed. Chicago: American Hospital Publishing, 1992.

Umbdenstock, R. J. Trustees and the integration of community health care. *Trustee* 46(5):14–17, May 1993.

Umbdenstock, R. J., and Hageman, W. M., editors. *Critical Readings for Hospital Trustees.* Chicago: American Hospital Publishing, 1991.

Unland, J. J. *The Trustee's Guide to Understanding Hospital Business Fundamentals.* Westchester, IL: Healthcare Financial Management Association, 1991.

Williams, J. B. Guidelines for managing integration. *Healthcare Forum Journal* 35(2):39–41, 44–47, Mar.–Apr. 1992.

Yee, D. K. Pass or fail? how to grade strategic process. *The Journal of Business Strategy* 11(3):10–14, May 1990.

Periodicals

American Hospital Association. *AHA News.*
This weekly newspaper published each Monday reports the most recent developments affecting hospitals, physicians, and the health care delivery system.

American Hospital Association. *Economic Trends.*
This quarterly newsletter provides subscribers with written analyses of hospital finances, utilization, and staffing trends.

American Hospital Publishing, Inc., an American Hospital Association company. *Hospitals & Health Networks.*
This semimonthly magazine for leaders of the health care field analyzes recent trends in collaborative health care delivery networks and patient-centered care, health care reform, and other complex health care delivery concerns and issues.

American Hospital Publishing, Inc. *Trustee.*
This monthly publication is the only magazine that exclusively covers the roles and responsibilities of hospital trustees. Many of the articles are written by trustees themselves.

Aspen Publishers, Inc. *Health Care Management Review.*
This quarterly publication for health care executives addresses a full range of concerns including financial development, quality assurance, staffing, and cost containment.

Aspen Publishers, Inc. *Hospital Strategy Report.*
This monthly newsletter concisely addresses issues of interest to health care executives and board members, including strategic planning, cost containment, retention, and recruitment.

Bader and Associates. *The Quality Letter for Healthcare Leaders.*
This newsletter focuses on health care quality issues and systems. Prepared specifically for trustees, it focuses on what boards need to know in this evolving subject area.

Ernst & Young. *Direct Connection.*
This biweekly newsletter provides health care executives with current information on federal and state regulatory and legislative activities.

Ernst & Young. *Health Care Briefing.*
This quarterly publication discusses topics of interest to health care executives, including regulatory and legislative matters, integrated systems, and quality.

Ernst & Young. *Health Care Tax Review.*
Published bimonthly, this review highlights current health care tax issues, including state and federal activities.

Terms You Need to Know

Accounting system: Methods and records established to identify, assemble, analyze, classify, record, and report an entity's transactions and to maintain accountability for related assets and liabilities (Source: American Institute of Certified Public Accountants, Statement of Auditing Standards No. 55, "Consideration of the Internal Control Structure in a Financial Statement Audit")

Affiliation: Formal combination of two or more health care organizations according to one of numerous organizational forms that maintains the identity of the preexisting organizations but allows for shared management functions

Balance sheet: Financial statement illustrating an entity's assets, liabilities, and net assets at a specific point in time

Base-case scenario: Forecast of an organization's outcomes assuming no change on the part of the organization, that is, a forecast of the impact of the external environment

Benchmark: Comparative performance or financial indicator considered to be an industry standard

Blended rate: Payment rate representing a combination, or blending, of different payment rates (for example, a combination of a federally determined rate and a hospital-specific rate)

Brainstorming: Group problem-solving technique that involves the spontaneous contribution of ideas from all members of the group

Business plan: Detailed, practical plan for implementing an organization's strategies and achieving an organization's goals over a relatively short period of time, usually about one year

Capitation: Method of payment for health services under which an individual or institutional provider is paid a fixed, per capita amount for each person served without regard to the actual number or nature of services provided

Case management: System of assessment, treatment planning, referral, and follow-up that ensures the provision of comprehensive and continuous service and the coordination of payment and reimbursement for care

Case mix: Categories of patients, classified by disease, procedure, method of payment, or other characteristics, in an institution at a given time, usually measured by counting or aggregating groups of patients sharing one or more characteristics

Certificate-of-need legislation: Legislation that requires health care organizations to apply for a certificate of approval from a state planning agency before constructing or modifying facilities, making major capital expenditures, or offering new or different services

Comparative performance analysis: Assessment of a health care organization's performance indicators against indicators of other area providers, industry averages, and so forth

Consolidation: Formal combination of two or more health care organizations into a new legal entity that has an identity separate from any of the preexisting organizations

Cost-based reimbursement: Payment by a third-party payer of the allowable costs incurred by a hospital in the provision of services to covered patients

Cost report: Cost analysis prepared by a health care provider as a basis for claiming reimbursable costs under third-party contracts

Day equivalents, inpatient: Sum of all inpatient service days, plus, over the same period, the volume of outpatient services expressed in units equivalent to inpatient service days

Demand forecasting: Process of projecting demand for health care services in a specific market for some future period of time, typically at least five years

Diagnosis-related group (DRG): Grouping of patients by diagnosis and treatment for purposes of reimbursement, specifically for Medicare reimbursement

Feasibility study: Independent evaluation of a facility's expansion or construction plan, including a report on the facility's financial forecast and a comprehensive economic and financial evaluation

Fee schedule: Price list for health care services rendered

Focal area: Major area of activity to be undertaken by an organization

Health maintenance organization (HMO): Organization that has management responsibility for providing comprehensive health care services on a prepaid basis to voluntarily enrolled persons within a designated population

Implementation schedule: Translation of strategies into specific operational priorities, timetables, and responsibilities

Inpatient: Person who receives medical or other health-related services while lodged in a hospital or other health care institution for at least one night

Intermediary: Blue Cross plan, private insurance company, or other public or private agency contracted by the federal government to pay claims under Medicare

Length of stay: Number of calendar days that elapse between an inpatient's admission and discharge

Liquidity support: Entity's available cash and investments to fund (if necessary) short-term debt requirements

Managed care: Health care provided under prepaid plans (such as health maintenance organizations and preferred provider organizations) or under various forms of direct employer intervention, with the goal of controlling the utilization and cost of health care services for participants in the plans

Market area: Geographic area from which the majority of a health care organization's patients come

Market channel: Health care organization's source of patients, which usually takes the form of physicians, health plans, or direct contracts

Market potential: Size of the total market an organization could capture in terms of dollars, type of care, and type of service need

Medicaid: Federally established (under Title XIX), state-administered, third-party payment program designed to pay for certain medical care provided to the indigent and medically indigent

Medicare: Federally established (under Title XVIII) third-party payment program administered by the Social Security Administration that pays for certain medical care provided to most persons age 65 and over and to some qualified persons under 65 (Part A covers hospital services; Part B covers physician services)

Merger: Formal combination of two or more health care organizations into a single new legal entity that may have the identity of one of the preexisting organizations

Objective: Concrete statement of a measurable target to be met in order to reach an organizational goal

Occupancy: Ratio of average daily census to the average number of beds maintained during the reporting period

Operating statistics: Entity's measures of operating activity, such as number of patient days or number of outpatient visits

Outpatient: Person who receives medical or other health-related services in a hospital or other health care institution but who is not lodged there

Outpatient visit: All services provided to an outpatient in the course of a single appearance in an outpatient or inpatient unit

Patient case mix: A measure of the diagnosis-specific makeup of a health care provider's patients

Patient origin: Geographic area of residence of patients

Payer: Entity (usually a business or the government) responsible for paying for insurance coverage or direct care

Performance indicator: Measure of organizational activity that can take the form of clinical outcomes, operations, quality, finances, and so forth

Physician group practice: Organization of two or more physicians, which may also include physician extenders

Physician–hospital integration: Combination of a hospital and a medical staff for the purpose of managing care, contracting, recruiting, planning, and so forth

Preferred provider organization (PPO): One of a variety of direct contractual relationships among hospitals, physicians, insurers, employers, or third-party administrators in which providers negotiate with group purchasers to provide health services for a defined population (such relationships typically include financial incentives for individual recipients of care to use contracting providers)

Prospective payment system: System that pays a predetermined and generally fixed payment per patient discharge category (generally per diagnosis-related group)

Provider: Health care organization or health care professional or group of organizations or professionals that provides health care services to patients

Provider network: Alliance of providers (physicians, hospitals, and outpatient and home health organizations) usually created for the purpose of managed care contracting

Reengineering: Redesign of an organization so that it delivers care differently in order to meet specific clinical and financial goals

Resource-based relative value scale (RBRVS): System used by Medicare to pay for physician services, based on the resources necessary to render services and the values of physician procedures

Self-insurance funding: Assets that are required to be placed in trust for self-insured claim deductibles under an arrangement with an insurance carrier

Service draw area: Area from which an organization is or could be attracting patients, usually defined geographically

Strategic assessment: Appraisal and analysis of the overall industry environment as well as the local market and the individual organization's position within that market

Strategic gap: Variance between future market and financial targets and the likely results an organization would achieve if it made no significant changes in its strategic position

Strategic plan: Comprehensive, far-ranging plan for fulfilling an organization's vision over a specified period of time, usually three to five years

Strategy: Statement of an organization's game plan for achieving certain goals and objectives

Third-party payer: An organization (usually an insurance company, prepayment plan, or government agency) that pays for health care services to a patient; most commonly used to refer to an agency that has an arrangement with a provider to care for a patient under a specific payment formula

Vision: What an organization wants to "look like" when its strategic plan is completely implemented

Appendix

A Finance Primer

In addition to overseeing the organization's strategic plan, it is the board's responsibility to monitor financial performance and to make sure a health care organization's financial resources are available and invested in a manner that supports the organization's strategic direction. Because of the health care field's unique characteristics, monitoring financial performance is perhaps the board's most challenging responsibility.

The purpose of this appendix is to help board members understand health care financial matters and to clarify their role in this complex area. Specifically, five aspects of the board's role in monitoring financial performance are discussed:

1. Developing a sound understanding of the common payment arrangements for health care services
2. Approving short- and long-range financial plans, goals, and measurement criteria that are linked to the organization's strategic direction, including budgets for operations, capital, and cash
3. Selecting methods of capital financing for major capital asset renovations, replacements, and additions or for new business ventures, programs, and services
4. Reviewing financial reports, operating statistics, and financial ratios on a regular basis to monitor financial performance relative to the strategic plan's financial goals
5. Monitoring the financial reporting process, which includes overseeing the independent audit of the organization's financial statements, monitoring information related to the organization's internal control structure, and overseeing the work of internal auditors

Understanding the Common Payment Arrangements

Health care entities receive payments for services from a variety of payers under a variety of payment plans. These diverse payment arrangements create complex financial considerations. If a board is to effectively address and monitor its health care organization's financial plans, goals, and measurement criteria, it must understand the typical payment arrangements of the major payers.

Payment for patient services comes from two types of sources: third-party payers (one or more) and patients. In some regions of the United States, third-party payers pay for as much as 90 percent of health care services rendered. Many third parties, such as Medicare, Medicaid, Blue Cross, other health insurance carriers, and managed care plans, pay providers on the basis of predetermined contractual rates or other methods rather than the provider's established rates.

Contractual Arrangements

Contractual arrangements with third-party payers are generally mandated or negotiated at levels that are lower than a provider's established charges. Any contract or arrangement between a provider and a payer based on anything other than the provider's established charges requires the provider to accept some financial risk. The nature and degree of this risk will vary depending on the unit of service and the basis for its payment. Table A-1 summarizes the risks and critical variables associated with different types of third-party payment arrangements or contracts.

Third-party payments to providers may end up being a combination of the contractual arrangements described in table A-1. For example, a hospital may have a discount arrangement with a commercial insurer (85 percent of charges), a per diem arrangement with Medicaid for inpatient services ($200 per day), a per case arrangement with Medicare for inpatient services ($500 per appendectomy), and a capitation arrangement with a health maintenance organization ($150 per member per month). The following sections discuss some of the major third-party payers for health care services and some common payment arrangements.

Medicare and Medicaid

Medicare is a federally administered program financed by payroll taxes as well as optional insurance premiums paid by beneficiaries for certain additional benefits. It covers a portion of hospital costs and physician fees for most persons 65 years old or older and eligible disabled persons. *Medicaid* programs were established to cover hospital costs and physician fees

Table A-1.   Risks by Contract Type

Payment Arrangement or Contract Type	Nature of Risk	Critical Variables
Discounted charges	Price[a]	Contribution margin[b]
Per diem	Price	Contribution margin
	Intensity[c]	Volume of ancillary services per patient Mix of days by service
Per case	Price	Contribution margin
	Intensity	Volume of ancillary services per patient Mix of days by service
	Severity[d]	Length of stay
Capitation	Price	Contribution margin
	Intensity	Volume of ancillary services per patient Mix of days by service
	Severity	Length of stay
	Frequency[e]	Admission rate Out-of-network claims costs

[a] *Contribution margin* is price less variable cost times volume.

[b] *Price risk* means that the provider is at risk that discounted prices will not cover variable costs and make an adequate contribution to overhead.

[c] *Intensity risk* means that the provider is at risk for correctly estimating average costs and the volume and mix of services provided each day. If actual intensity (volume and cost of services) is greater than anticipated, the provider will lose money.

[d] *Severity risk* means that the provider is at risk if the total cost of services required by a patient exceeds the revenue received for that patient. Payment is an average flat price per discharge category, regardless of length of stay and volume and cost of services provided.

[e] *Frequency risk* means that the provider is at risk for the overall use rates of enrollees because the provider assumes the obligation to provide all medical services required by enrollees (as defined by a covered benefits list) for a flat payment per enrollee, per month.

for low-income families and needy individuals. Both Medicare and Medicaid contract with providers and pay them directly for services rendered to beneficiaries.

Before 1983, Medicare paid hospitals for the costs they incurred in treating Medicare beneficiaries by determining allowable costs under reimbursement principles defined by Medicare. In 1983, Medicare instituted a prospective payment system (PPS) that radically changed the basis of hospital payment. Under PPS, most inpatient hospital services are paid on the basis of a prospectively determined rate for each discharge. This rate is based on a patient's assignment to a diagnosis-related group (DRG). Referring to table A-1, Medicare's DRG payment is an example of a per case payment. Generally, the actual hospital charges and costs incurred in providing services to a patient have no effect on the amount of the DRG payment under PPS.

The 1983 change from cost-based payments to prospective payments for most inpatient services was just the beginning of a long series of changes in the Medicare payment system. Over time, cost-based payments for certain outpatient services, inpatient capital costs, and other services have been replaced by prospective payment methods, fee schedules, defined blended rates, and other payment systems. The payment system for physician services is changing from the traditional fee-for-service system to a *resource-based relative value scale* (RBRVS), which provides physician payments based on relative value units and fee schedules. If a new hospital program or service is expected to involve significant Medicare reimbursement, the hospital's board should understand the basis of Medicare payment and challenge its adequacy.

Under the Medicaid program, each state establishes its own payment program and selects specific coverage options. States pay providers using a variety of methods, including discounted charges and per diem, per case, and cost-based payment systems.

Traditional Insurance Programs and Managed Care Plans

Traditional health insurance programs usually represent between 10 and 30 percent of a provider's source of revenue and typically pay the provider on the basis of established rates or a discount arrangement. Far more prevalent, however, are managed care plans, which represent a growing share of providers' revenues in many parts of the United States. Health maintenance organizations (HMOs) and preferred provider organizations (PPOs) are the most popular of the many types of managed care programs.

Managed care programs provide comprehensive health care services to their enrollees either directly or through contractual arrangements with other providers. Each enrollee prepays a monthly premium to the managed care plan regardless of the volume of health care services used. Medical services are delivered by health care providers who are partners or employees of the plan or by providers under contractual arrangements with the plan.

Managed care plans with large numbers of enrollees can funnel patients to the providers that have contracted with them. With their bargaining power, managed care plans negotiate contracts with providers under the contract payment methods described in table A-1. Because of the financial risks and critical variables highlighted in table A-1, health care providers involved in managed care contracts must carefully project patient volume, know their costs of providing services, and monitor the financial and operational results of their contracts.

Self-Pay Revenues

A patient with no third-party coverage is a *self-pay* patient. For each service provided, the patient pays the provider's established charges. Self-pay revenues include payments made by a patient as part of deductible or coinsurance arrangements required by third-party payers.

Charity Care

Charity care is provided by health care organizations that have a policy to provide health care services free of charge to individuals who meet certain financial criteria. However, it is often hard to distinguish between charity care and bad debts. Generally, bad debts result from the unwillingness of a patient to pay, whereas charity service is provided to a patient with a demonstrated inability to pay.[1] Charity care, therefore, is not expected to result in cash flow to a provider and is not recognized as revenue or receivables in a provider's financial statements. However, board members who are concerned about their health care organization's responsibility to provide charity care and community benefits may request charity care information from management. Such information on charity services provided can be measured on the basis of charges, costs, or appropriate statistics.

Other Operating Revenue and Nonoperating Gains

Although most provider revenues are derived from patient services, other sources of revenue are common and often represent significant funds for health care organizations. These sources of operating revenue and nonoperating gains include tuition from educational programs, voluntary charitable contributions, tax support and other subsidies, investment income, and income from other miscellaneous sources. Health care organizations with significant endowments or support from other sources consider these amounts when formulating financial plans and goals.

Health Care Budgeting

With a basic understanding of the common payment arrangements for health care services described in the preceding sections, the board will be prepared to consider budgeting and other financial aspects of the strategic planning process. A *budget* is the financial expression of a health care organization's strategic plan and an important tool in allocating an organization's scarce resources to achieve the goals of its plan. The budget directs the implementation of planning decisions and monitors the results of those decisions.

If the budget is to be an effective tool, both the board and management must take part in the budget development process and monitor the budget's financial results. A solid strategic plan is likely to fail without the support of a budget infrastructure. The budget should perform several tasks, including the following:

- Provide a plan for operations, cash, and capital to achieve goals
- Provide measurable performance standards
- Identify unexpected changes in operations and cash so that adjustments can be made

An effective budget process is not an exercise that takes place only once a year; it is an ongoing process of accumulating and comparing data, investigating variances, modifying performance, and revising plans. Figure A-1 illustrates the continuous flow of information that makes up the budget process.

The operating budget, capital budget, and cash flow budget are three types of budgets that support a health care organization's strategic direction in different but interrelated ways. They each fulfill specific functions in the financial planning process and should be prepared and monitored regularly.

The Operating Budget

A health care organization's operating budget generally covers one fiscal year, and its fundamental components are patient service volume and other utilization forecasts, expense estimates, and revenue projections. The overall operating budget is a summary of the more-detailed budgets prepared for each of an organization's departments or divisions.

Figure A-1. The Budget Process

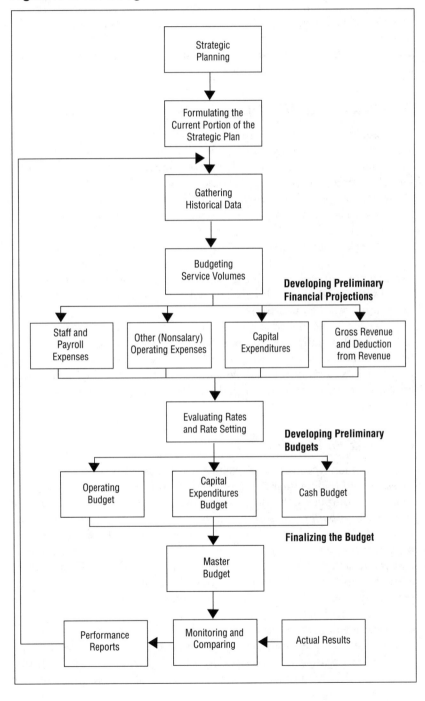

The operating budget's revenue projections and expense estimates are developed on the basis of service volume projections. If actual service volume falls short of projections, then the impact of this shortfall on the revenue and expense components of the operating budget must be assessed, and action must be taken (if possible) to minimize the impact on the organization's financial goals.

Fixed versus Flexible Operating Budgets

Fixed budgets help monitor operating results during the budget year. They are usually adjusted only when major changes in operations or budget assumptions occur. Flexible budgets are adjusted periodically as actual service volume and cost data become available. These data are used to revise budget projections throughout the year. Flexible budgets allow managers to isolate the impact of differences in volume from other trends.

Preparing a flexible budget requires analysis of an organization's variable (that is, volume-dependent) and fixed-cost components. As projected service volumes are adjusted on the basis of actual operating results, the variable portion of operating expenses is increased or decreased to correspond to the new volume levels. The impact on revenues and the operating margin can then be determined.

Flexible budgeting requires some effort, but it is worthwhile because it enables an organization to take timely corrective action to achieve its financial goals despite service volume shortfalls. In addition, when compared to a fixed budget, a flexible budget is a more meaningful yardstick by which to measure departmental efficiency and productivity throughout the year.

Case Mix and Product Lines

Like manufacturing companies, many health care entities anticipate their revenues and budget their resource needs on the basis of product-specific inputs and outputs, defining and measuring their products in aggregate terms such as *patient days, admissions, discharges,* and *outpatient visits.* Although these measures help indicate overall production levels, an organization's patient demographics and the various health care needs of its patients should be considered in the budgeting process. These considerations, along with the entity's patient case mix, are important when projecting net revenues and estimating operating expense requirements in this time of contractual payment arrangements.

Service volume forecasts that consider both service quantity and case mix intensity are ideal for budget planning and control purposes. In comparison to forecasts that consider only service quantity, they provide better estimates of the patient care resources that will be expended and the revenues that will be received from payers who make payments on a per case basis.

The Capital Budget

The *capital budget* establishes guidelines for the replacement, renovation, and acquisition of new buildings and equipment under the strategic plan. The capital budget generally spans three years, although an annual review and update is recommended so that the health care organization's most current financial position and financing capacity can be considered before any significant capital commitments are made.

The Cash Flow Budget

The period covered by the cash flow budget usually parallels that of the operating budget. The *cash flow budget* is a forecast of future cash receipts and cash disbursements. Even though a health care organization may budget for positive operating income for the year, the timing of cash transactions may not necessarily accommodate the organization's working capital needs. The cash flow budget estimates cash balances at interim periods throughout the year so that plans can be made to maximize earnings on idle funds and identify periods of cash needs.

Capital Financing

Planning for a health care organization's capital asset or new program needs must begin with the organization's long-range strategic plan for health care programs and services. The strategic plan provides the framework within which management and the medical staff identify and recommend capital asset purchases and program development. The board, through its involvement with the strategic planning process, will be aware of these projects and priorities and will share the responsibility for financing them. The following sections discuss the board's role in capital financing, which includes selecting a method of financing and determining the organization's maximum debt level.

Selecting a Method of Financing

Some health care organizations have funds resulting from charitable pledge drives, endowment fund earnings, and/or operations that enable them to purchase capital assets and/or develop new programs. However, few organizations are in a position to purchase capital assets or develop new programs without some form of borrowing such as loan arrangements, leasing, or capital-raising activities (for example, partnership formation or joint venturing).

Health care entities can usually access the wide variety of financing vehicles that are available to corporate entities. These include long- and short-term financing vehicles and taxable and tax-exempt forms of financing. The basic types of loan arrangements and their characteristics are summarized in tables A-2 and A-3.

Tax-exempt bonds, a popular form of long-term financing, are made available to health care entities through state and local health facilities financing authorities. This form of financing is fairly complex but has several advantages, including generally lower interest rates, that cannot be found in other financing arrangements.

The board should recognize that leasing is an alternative form of debt financing. Leasing should be given the same kind of evaluation by the board as other forms of debt financing. Too often, leasing costs are viewed as an element of the operating budget, and leasing decisions are left to department managers.

The Long- and Short-Term Debt Markets

As illustrated in tables A-2 and A-3, each type of financing arrangement in the long- and short-term debt markets has advantages and disadvantages. Further complicating the evaluation of these arrangements are the many different lenders and market factors that result in rapidly changing interest rates and unpredictable fund availability. Just as it is important to plan for capital asset or new project needs, it is also important to plan for the financing of those needs at the same time. The factors that should be considered in selecting a form of debt financing include the following:

- Needs and borrowing ability
  - Cost of a project and the amount of financing required to meet that cost
  - Need for interim financing during the period of construction of a capital asset
  - Need for working capital financing during start-up of a new program
  - Ability to assume additional debt *(debt capacity)*
  - Ability to borrow, as affected by legal restrictions, market conditions, and an organization's credit standing
- Costs and effects on operations
  - Loan interest rate and the amount of fees and other costs to obtain a loan
  - Credit enhancement options, such as lines and letters of credit and bond insurance that lower interest rates

Table A-2.   Long-Term Debt Market

	Sources for Obtaining Funds	Amount of Financing Available	Debt Maturity and Prepayment	Financing Cost	Primary Advantages	Primary Disadvantages
Tax-Exempt Bonds	Investment bankers	100% of costs	Generally 20 to 30 years; prepayment after 10 years	Generally lowest interest rates because of tax-exempt feature	Lower equity requirements; generally 1% to 3% lower interest rates; flexibility of repayment period	Less flexibility to prepay and generally more operating restrictions
Taxable Bonds	Investment bankers	100% of costs	10 to 15 years, usually with large final payment; prepayment flexible	Generally 1% to 3% above tax-exempt rates	More flexible loan terms	Higher interest costs and equity requirements
Mortgages	Banks or savings and loan institutions	Set by lender and regulation, usually 50% to 75% of costs	Generally 15 to 25 years; prepayment varies with lender	Generally 1% to 3% above tax-exempt rates	Shorter length of time to arrange loan	Higher interest costs and equity requirements
Federal Government Loan Programs	Mortgage bankers or banks	90% of estimated replacement costs	25 years; prepayment of 15% per year without penalty	Generally 1% to 3% above tax-exempt rates	More accessible to high-risk borrowers	Higher interest costs, longer time to arrange loan, and compliance requirements
Leases	Banks, leasing companies, and equipment vendors	100% of costs	Debt maturity and prepayment vary	Significantly above other rates	Greater ability to take advantage of new equipment and technology	Higher total financing costs

Table A-3. Short-Term Debt Market

	Sources for Obtaining Funds	Debt Maturity and Prepayment	Financing Cost	Security	Primary Advantages	Primary Disadvantages
Demand Bonds	Investment bankers	1 to 30 years—however, purchaser may demand payment within days of notice; dealer may remarket bonds on "best efforts" basis; issuer may prepay	Variable	Line or letter of credit, bond insurance, or high-grade collateral	Flexible repayment period	Need liquidity support if demand is made and bond cannot be remarketed
Tender Bonds	Investment bankers	1 to 30 years—however, issuer may convert into fixed-rate long-term debt; purchaser may put bonds back to issuer; dealer may remarket bonds on "best efforts" basis	Variable	Line or letter of credit, bond insurance, or high-grade collateral	Issuer may convert bonds into fixed-rate debt	Need liquidity support if bond is put back to issuer and bond cannot be remarketed
Tax-Exempt Commercial Paper	Investment bankers	1 to 270 days, but typically 90 days; purchaser cannot demand payment; issuer cannot prepay	Fixed	Line of credit	Less collateral required	Need liquidity support; available only to high-net-worth organizations
Line of Credit	Banks	Usually 1 year	Generally higher	Limited	May borrow when needed; limited collateral requirements	Bank may cancel line if creditworthiness changes; fees for unused portion of line
Leases	Banks, leasing companies, and equipment vendors	Debt maturity and prepayment vary	Significantly above other rates	Property leased	Greater ability to take advantage of new equipment and technology	Higher total financing cost

— Length of time required to obtain a loan
— Restrictions that a debt will place on an organization's operations
— Information concerning an organization's operations that must be provided to obtain a loan
— Amount and type of assets that must be mortgaged, as well as the assets required by lenders for debt service contingency and other reserves

The board and management must weigh each of the preceding factors to determine which method of financing is best for their organization.

Financial Feasibility Studies

If the board and management decide to issue bonds to finance capital spending, a financial feasibility study may be a part of the financing package. Financial feasibility studies have become important—and often mandatory—documents for any public sale of bonds to fund health care facility expansion or new construction. The study is usually less essential when debt is privately placed because of the lender's technical and practical ability to conduct its own evaluation based on its specific guidelines. However, any potential lender values a well-prepared study presenting extensive financial material in a concise and logical manner, whether the material relates to tax-exempt or taxable debt and whether the debt is publicly sold or privately placed.

A *health care feasibility study* is an independent evaluation of the expected future outcome(s) of a health care facility's plans and programs. This study includes an accountant's examination report on the facility's financial forecast and a comprehensive economic and financial evaluation. The feasibility study focuses on the facility's cash-generating capacity and assesses the adequacy of cash flows to meet the facility's financial needs. Specifically, the health care feasibility study analyzes the following elements:

- *Strategic plan:* The facility's health care role and future plans in the defined service area, including demographic and economic factors that affect future utilization in the service area
- *Market area facilities:* The potential impact of ongoing or proposed expansion, modernization, and/or program plan changes of other service area facilities
- *Medical staff:* Medical staff attitudes toward and degree of support for the proposed expansion and modernization program
- *Operations:* Changes in operational matters such as third-party payer agreements, staffing requirements, and salary and nonsalary costs
- *Financing:* The timing, cost, and financing assumptions of the program

Although most feasibility studies refer to *debt service coverage,* which is of interest to bond purchasers, the health care feasibility study report generally expresses its conclusion in terms of the adequacy of total cash flows and the reasonableness of assumptions related to the facility's forecasted cash flows.

Rating agencies generally require a feasibility study before rating bonds, and bond purchasers use the study as a basis for deciding whether to buy a particular bond issue. All parties in the financing program expect the study to be detailed, thorough, and rigorous. Although hospital management is often capable of preparing a feasibility study, the study has evolved into a third-party evaluation of the facility's financial and operational viability and requires the independence and objectivity of an outside consultant.

Debt Capacity

Determining a health care organization's maximum amount of debt is a key responsibility of its board. Although the board may commit funds from past, current, and future operations for capital spending, the board and management must decide how much their organization can safely borrow and repay. To use a lender's term, this maximum level of debt is often called the organization's *debt capacity.*

When a lender determines an organization's debt capacity, it considers a variety of economic and other factors in order to evaluate the organization's operations; expected program, service, and facility changes; and present and expected financial strength. Some of the nonfinancial factors that are generally evaluated include the following:

- The organization's potential market and the organization's existing and expected market share
- The organization's ability to attract patients based on medical staff characteristics, the organization's range of services, and the condition and location of its facilities
- The effectiveness of the organization's strategic plan and budgeting process
- The level of community support for the organization
- The effectiveness of the organization's board and management

The financial factors considered by lenders evaluating an organization's debt capacity include the following:

- Anticipated cash flows from operations
- The organization's debt coverage ratio
- The ratio of debt service requirements to net operating revenue

- The level of present and proposed debt compared to the value of the entity's net assets (the debt-to-equity ratio)

Although lenders and rating agencies use some benchmarks for evaluating debt capacity, a health care organization's unique situation may require specific discussions with the lenders and agencies. Discussions and meetings among lenders and agencies and management should result in decisions and conclusions that leave board members confident in their organization's ability to service a particular debt.

Other Financing Alternatives

Because of the continuing financial and operational pressures on health care providers, many entities have expanded programs and obtained capital assets through collaborations with other health care providers. Affiliations, ventures, partnerships, and other business combinations have become popular means of financing and expanding health care services. For example, if two hospitals need an expensive capital asset but neither has the financial resources to secure the asset at a reasonable cost, a venture or other contractual arrangement to acquire and operate the asset may be an effective method to expand services. With many providers seeking opportunities to network their health care services with other providers, these types of affiliations and collaborations will present the board with alternatives to traditional financing arrangements.

Reviewing Financial Reports, Operating Statistics, and Financial Ratios

Financial analysis is an important tool for monitoring a health care organization's performance in relation to the financial goals of its strategic plan. Such analysis may identify trends that confirm movement toward financial goals or that suggest a need for corrective action. Financial trend analysis generally relies on the use of financial ratios. A *financial ratio* expresses the relationship of one financial item to another in a simple mathematical form. Comparing the ratios of one entity to the ratios of other entities or to the entity's past values is an easy and quick process.

The health care field has developed a wide variety of operating statistics and financial ratios that can provide board members with comprehensive, quantitative information about their organization's financial and operational status and trends. To help ensure an understanding of these financial ratios and statistics, board members should review their organization's basic financial statements.

A sample statement of revenue and expenses, a sample balance sheet, and a sample statement of cash flows are illustrated in figures A-2, A-3, and A-4, respectively. These samples provide references for the concepts to be covered in the following sections. In addition, figure A-2 includes commonly used statistical information. Because these figures are only examples, they do not reflect the possible operational combinations of a diversified health care provider, and they may not reflect the format or level of detail that individual board members may need. It is the board's responsibility to work with management to determine what information board members need to fulfill their responsibilities.

It should be noted that the American Institute of Certified Public Accountants (AICPA) is currently considering revisions to its *Audit and Accounting Guide: Audits of Providers of Health Care Services* (the Guide).[2] The Guide is the central document governing health care accounting and reporting practices. Forthcoming revisions to the Guide, required by the issuance of two Financial Accounting Standards Board statements in June 1993 that affected not-for-profit entities, are expected to reflect changes in financial statement display and accounting for contributions. For this appendix's purposes, the financial statements in figures A-2, A-3, and A-4 are based on the current Guide. Revisions to the Guide are not expected to have a significant impact on the topics discussed in this appendix.

Statement of Revenue and Expenses and Operating Statistics

By reviewing the statement of revenue and expenses (see figure A-2), board members can determine whether their organization is achieving its planned operating margin and whether any corrective action is necessary to ensure that the organization meets the strategic plan's financial requirements. The statement of revenue and expenses is most useful when reviewed with key operating or utilization statistics in mind. The key statistics that are usually part of this review are inpatient days, outpatient visits, percentage occupancy, admissions, discharges, ancillary procedures, full-time equivalent (FTE) personnel, and services provided by case type and payer classification.

As noted in chapter 1, the financial incentives for a health care provider that has contracted to provide health care services for a fixed fee to large population groups are dramatically different from those of a provider working under traditional payment arrangements. Rather than being driven to increase volumes of admissions or procedures, a provider paid under a capitation arrangement will work to keep its populations as healthy as possible and drive down utilization rates. A statistic measuring the level of health care contracted under capitation arrangements would be particularly helpful to providers in such arrangements. The number of

Figure A-2. Sample Statement of Revenue and Expenses (Unrestricted Net Assets) and Operating Statistics

	Current Year Actual	Current Year Budgeted	Prior Year Actual
Operating statistics:			
Average beds available	220	225	225
Patient days	40,150	42,705	44,348
Percent occupancy	50	52	54
Average length of stay (days)	7.2	7.5	7.5
Outpatient visits	36,390	33,360	30,330
Net patient service revenue:			
Inpatient	$44,000,000	$46,000,000	$45,000,000
Outpatient	13,100,000	12,000,000	10,000,000
Total	$57,100,000	$58,000,000	$55,000,000
Capitation revenue	$ 3,000,000	$ 2,700,000	$ 2,600,000
Other operating revenue	3,100,000	3,300,000	3,000,000
Total operating revenue	$63,200,000	$64,000,000	$60,600,000
Operating expenses:			
Salaries and wages	$28,200,000	$28,500,000	$27,000,000
Employee benefits	3,400,000	3,250,000	3,100,000
Supplies and other expenses	17,700,000	17,550,000	16,500,000
Purchased services	4,950,000	4,750,000	4,500,000
Bad debts	1,200,000	1,500,000	1,300,000
Depreciation	4,200,000	4,200,000	4,300,000
Interest	3,150,000	3,200,000	3,100,000
Total operating expenses	$62,800,000	$62,950,000	$59,800,000
Income from operations	$ 400,000	$ 1,050,000	800,000
Nonoperating gains	350,000	450,000	400,000
Revenue and gains in excess of expenses	$ 750,000	$ 1,500,000	$ 1,200,000

covered lives and the per member per month (PMPM) payment are informative statistics for providers with significant capitation arrangements. A board member's understanding of the different types of payment contracts is critical to his or her accurate interpretation of such statistics.

Utilization statistics should be compared with budgeted amounts for the same period and actual performance during the prior period. Trends in admissions, inpatient days, average lengths of stay, and occupancy percentages are indicators of changes in the provider's market. Upward or downward trends may have been anticipated in the budget and therefore confirm that the provider's budget expectations are on target. Unexpected adverse changes in utilization, however, may indicate potential obstacles to meeting financial goals. There are many possible reasons for a decline in utilization, including the loss of a major payer contract or problems in

Figure A-3.   Sample Balance Sheet

	Current Year Actual	Current Year Budgeted	Prior Year Actual
Assets			
Current assets:			
Cash and cash equivalents	$ 2,000,000	$ 3,000,000	$ 2,500,000
Patient accounts receivable, net	11,000,000	10,500,000	10,000,000
Supplies	800,000	730,000	750,000
Other current assets	200,000	220,000	200,000
Total current assets	$14,000,000	$14,450,000	$13,450,000
Assets whose use is limited or restricted:			
By board for capital improvements	$ 5,000,000	$ 5,500,000	$ 5,000,000
Under malpractice funding arrangement—			
held by trustee	1,900,000	1,800,000	1,500,000
Under indenture agreement—held			
by trustee	2,600,000	2,600,000	2,700,000
By donors for specific purposes	750,000	700,000	1,000,000
By donors for permanent endowments	4,750,000	4,800,000	4,700,000
	$15,000,000	$15,400,000	$14,900,000
Property and equipment, net	45,800,000	46,000,000	45,000,000
Other assets	1,250,000	1,200,000	1,100,000
Total assets	$76,050,000	$77,050,000	$74,450,000
Liabilities and net assets			
Current liabilities:			
Accounts payable	$ 3,700,000	$ 3,500,000	$ 3,500,000
Accrued expenses	2,600,000	2,500,000	2,500,000
Estimated third-party settlement	750,000	800,000	1,000,000
Current portion of long-term debt	1,200,000	1,400,000	1,000,000
Total current liabilities	$ 8,250,000	$ 8,200,000	$ 8,000,000
Long-term debt, less current portion	$40,800,000	$41,000,000	$40,000,000
Estimated malpractice costs	$ 700,000	$ 800,000	$ 700,000
Net assets:			
Unrestricted	$20,600,000	$21,350,000	$19,850,000
Temporarily restricted	950,000	900,000	1,200,000
Permanently restricted	4,750,000	4,800,000	4,700,000
Total net assets	$26,300,000	$27,050,000	$25,750,000
Total liabilities and net assets	$76,050,000	$77,050,000	$74,450,000

the practice of a key medical staff member. The board and management must act appropriately to address adverse utilization trends.

Revenue and expense items should be analyzed not only in comparison with utilization statistics, but also in comparison with budgeted amounts and actual prior period amounts, as shown in figure A-2. This analysis might indicate to board members that outpatient visits and revenue are increasing at rates greater than budget and much greater than in the prior year. Additionally, the same analysis might indicate that inpa-

Figure A-4.   Sample Statement of Cash Flows (Unrestricted Net Assets)

	Current Year Actual	Current Year Budgeted	Prior Year Actual
Cash flows from operating activities and gains:			
Revenue and gains in excess of expenses	$ 750,000	$1,500,000	$1,200,000
Adjustments to reconcile revenue and gains in excess of expenses to net cash provided by operating activities and gains:			
Depreciation	4,200,000	4,200,000	4,300,000
Provision for bad debts	1,200,000	1,500,000	1,300,000
Increase in patient accounts receivable	(2,200,000)	(2,000,000)	(1,500,000)
Increase in supplies and other assets	(50,000)	0	(100,000)
Increase in accounts payable and accrued expenses	300,000	0	100,000
Decrease in estimated third-party settlement	(250,000)	(200,000)	(50,000)
Increase in medical malpractice costs	0	100,000	150,000
Increase in other assets	(150,000)	(100,000)	(50,000)
Net cash provided by operating activities and gains	$3,800,000	$5,000,000	$5,350,000
Cash flows from investing activities:			
Purchase of property and equipment	($5,000,000)	($5,200,000)	($4,000,000)
Cash invested in assets whose use is limited	(300,000)	(700,000)	(500,000)
Net cash used by investing activities	($5,300,000)	($5,900,000)	($4,500,000)
Cash flows from financing activities:			
Repayment of long-term debt	($1,000,000)	($1,000,000)	($ 800,000)
Borrowings of long-term debt	2,000,000	2,400,000	1,000,000
Net cash provided by financing activities	$1,000,000	$1,400,000	$ 200,000
Net increase (decrease) in cash	(500,000)	500,000	1,050,000
Cash at beginning of year	2,500,000	2,500,000	1,450,000
Cash at end of year	$2,000,000	$3,000,000	$2,500,000

tient admissions, occupancy, and revenue will be adversely affected by this greater-than-expected move toward outpatient services. In such a scenario, the board might ask whether appropriate staffing adjustments and changes in support functions have been made to address a significant increase in outpatient services. By performing a comparative analysis of financial and statistical data and by asking penetrating questions to gain a thorough understanding of the situation, the board can work with management to assess the impact of unexpected variations in revenue and expenses on the organization's planned performance and determine whether corrective actions are needed.

Statement of Financial Position: Balance Sheet

A health care organization's statement of financial position, or *balance sheet* (see figure A-3, p. 114), is another valuable tool for monitoring performance. Although a health care organization's balance sheet is similar to that of other industries, a few differences warrant discussion. Unlike most other industries, not-for-profit health care entities generally have "restricted assets" and "assets whose use is limited" on the balance sheet.

Restricted assets are funds that are restricted for a specific purpose by a donor or grantor. For example, a donor may contribute funds to a health care organization for a construction project (temporarily restricted funds) or for an endowment (permanently restricted funds). These restricted assets are used only for the purpose identified by the donor and are not available for general operating purposes. Other types of assets with limited use include the following:

- Assets set aside by the board for identified purposes (sometimes referred to as *board-designated assets*). Board-designated assets could be funds set aside for a construction program or to initiate a new service. The board retains control over the assets and may, at its discretion, use them for other purposes. (The *board-designated assets* caption on the balance sheet may be discontinued under expected revisions to the Guide.)
- Proceeds of debt issues and funds deposited with a trustee that are limited to use in accordance with the requirements of an indenture or similar agreement.
- Assets limited to use for identified purposes through an agreement between the organization and an outside party other than a donor. For example, many health care entities have assets set aside under self-insurance funding arrangements.

Just as with the statement of revenue and expenses, the board can use comparative historical and budgeted balance sheets along with other supplemental information to monitor performance. In addition, the board can evaluate whether funds are available to meet the needs of the strategic plan. More specifically, after reviewing the financial requirements of the strategic plan, the board might ask whether funds are available to adequately finance major capital asset additions or new business ventures. If the health care organization has a large amount of funds that are restricted or limited as to use and insufficient available funds, then the financing of new projects will be a critical concern for the board. Sources of new-project financing might include tax-exempt bonds or other vehicles, as discussed earlier in this appendix, or funds generated from operations, as illustrated in the statement of cash flows. (See figure A-4, p. 115.)

Statement of Cash Flows

Although a health care organization's statement of cash flows, like its balance sheet, is similar to those used by other industries, a brief comment about its importance in monitoring financial performance is appropriate. Normally prepared annually or as part of a forecast for a new project, the *statement of cash flows* illustrates the net cash provided by or used by an organization's operating activities, investing activities, and financing activities. The statement provides board members with answers to the most basic question of a business enterprise—how does the entity generate and use cash? For significant new projects and service programs, management should prepare a statement of cash flow and consider various funding and operational viability matters with the board. In addition, by comparing actual cash flow performance to the budget or expected cash flow, the board can better assist management in taking appropriate action to achieve performance objectives.

Financial Ratios

In addition to reviewing comparative financial statements and key statistics, board members can utilize financial ratio analysis to obtain valuable information about their organization's financial position and operations. Financial ratio analysis can identify potentially negative trends, provide information about financial capacity (creditworthiness), and monitor the effectiveness of vital financial areas such as patient accounts receivable. Ratio analysis can also highlight industry trends and provide a basis for comparisons with other entities.

Ratio analysis allows health care organizations to compare their current financial results to their results from prior periods, to the results of other organizations in the area, and to industrywide averages. When a ratio seems out of line, an investigation may be warranted. However, the board should be careful not to draw hasty conclusions. Unusual accounting methods, hospital sizes, and operating environments can produce ratios that are not comparable to those of other hospitals. Significant events, for example, the addition of a new service or hospital resizing, can create changes in an entity's financial trends that might be misinterpreted.

There are four major categories of financial ratios:

1. *Liquidity ratios* measure the ability of an organization to meet its short-term obligations.
2. *Profitability ratios* measure an organization's ability to generate a return from operations.
3. *Leverage* or *capital structure ratios* measure an organization's ability to meet its long-term obligations and financial requirements.

4. *Turnover* or *activity ratios* measure an organization's ability to gener-
    ate net operating revenue in relation to various assets.

Table A-4 (pp. 120–21) provides calculations for and explanations of many
commonly used financial ratios. Health care board members, managers,
financial advisors, bond-rating agencies, and rate review organizations
use these ratios in their review of an entity's financial performance.

Monitoring the Financial Reporting Process

As it monitors an organization's financial performance, the board has
several key responsibilities that relate to the financial reporting process.
These responsibilities include overseeing the independent audit of the
entity's financial statements and internal control structure, as well as overseeing the internal audit function.

Independent Audit

Perhaps the board's most visible role in the financial reporting process is
its participation in the annual audit of the entity's financial statements,
including the selection of independent auditors. The independent auditors examine the financial statements to determine whether, in their opinion, the statements represent fairly and in all material respects the
organization's financial position, results of operations, and cash flows in
conformity with generally accepted accounting principles. When it selects
independent auditors, the board should ask many questions, including
the following:

- Is the auditing firm independent?
- What is the firm's health care industry expertise?
- Who will be assigned to the audit, and what are his or her or their
  qualifications and health care industry expertise?
- How much will the partner participate in the audit?
- What other professional services, for example, tax, consulting, or merg-
  ers and acquisitions assistance, are available from the firm?
- What are the firm's estimated fees, and how will differences between
  actual and estimated fees be handled?

During the annual audit, the board should ask independent auditors
about the audit's scope, approach, and results. Independent auditors usually supplement their report on an organization's financial statements with
a separate management letter covering their observations of the internal
control structure and recommendations. These observations often cover

financial, operational, and administrative matters. The board should consider asking the following questions when reviewing audit results with independent auditors:

- Will you issue an "unqualified opinion"?
- What significant estimates, for example, estimates of receivable allowances or Medicare program settlement amounts, were necessary in preparing the financial statements? Was the accounting treatment conservative or liberal?
- Were unusual transactions noted?
- Were there disagreements with management on accounting and reporting issues?
- Were there changes in accounting policies?
- What were your findings in high-risk audit areas?
- Were there significant deficiencies in the design or functioning of the internal control structure?
- What significant findings are reported in the management letter?

Although independent auditors work with management, they are generally engaged by and directly responsible to the board. The AICPA's code of ethics requires independent auditors to be completely independent of the organizations they audit. This requirement makes the auditors a valuable resource to the board as the board evaluates and monitors the adequacy of the organization's internal control structure and the accuracy of the organization's financial information.

Internal Control Structure

As part of its oversight role in the financial reporting process, the board acts as an interrogator, asking management and independent and internal auditors questions that will help determine whether the organization has controls that adequately safeguard its assets and whether the organization's financial statements "tell it like it is." With a basic understanding of the internal control structure, the board can direct its questions to the areas where problems are most likely to occur in the financial reporting process.

According to the AICPA, an organization's *internal control structure* consists of the policies and procedures established to provide reasonable assurance that specific organizational objectives will be achieved.[3] Although an organization's internal control structure may include a wide variety of objectives and related policies and procedures, not all of them may be relevant to an audit of the organization's financial statements. Consequently, only relevant objectives, policies, and procedures should be considered by the independent auditor.

Table A-4. Financial Ratios

Financial Ratio	Equation	Data Source[a]
Liquidity:		
1. Current ratio	$$\frac{\text{Current Assets}}{\text{Current Liabilities}}$$	AFS
2. Days of revenue in patient accounts receivable	$$\frac{\text{Net Patient Accounts Receivable}}{\text{Net Patient Service Revenue} \div 365}$$	AFS
3. Days cash on hand	$$\frac{\text{Cash + Short-Term Investments}}{(\text{Operating Expenses - Depreciation}) \div 365}$$	AFS
4. Average payment period	$$\frac{\text{Current Liabilities}}{(\text{Operating Expenses - Depreciation}) \div 365}$$	AFS
Profitability:		
5. Operating margin	$$\frac{\text{Operating Revenue - Operating Expenses}}{\text{Operating Revenue}}$$	AFS
6. Return on equity	$$\frac{\text{Revenue and Gains in Excess of Expenses and Losses}}{\text{Equity or Net Assets}}$$	AFS
7. Return on assets	$$\frac{\text{Revenue and Gains in Excess of Expenses and Losses}}{\text{Total Assets}}$$	AFS
Leverage or Capital Structure:		
8. Debt-to-equity or leverage ratio	$$\frac{\text{Long-Term Debt}}{\text{Equity or Net Assets}}$$	AFS
9. Debt service coverage ratio	$$\frac{\text{Cash Flow}^{b} + \text{Interest Expense}}{\text{Principal Payment + Interest Expense}}$$	AFS, OD
10. Cash flow to total debt ratio	$$\frac{\text{Cash Flow}^{b}}{\text{Total Liabilities}}$$	AFS, OD
Turnover or Activity:		
11. Average age of plant	$$\frac{\text{Accumulated Depreciation}}{\text{Depreciation Expense}}$$	AFS
12. Total asset turnover	$$\frac{\text{Total Operating Revenue}}{\text{Total Assets}}$$	AFS
13. Working capital turnover ratio	$$\frac{\text{Net Operating Revenue}}{\text{Total Current Assets - Total Current Liabilities}}$$	AFS

[a] *AFS* stands for audited financial statements; *OD* stands for other entity data.
[b] *Cash flow* is revenue and gains in excess of expenses and losses plus expenses not requiring cash (for example, depreciation, amortization, and other deferred items).

Table A-4. Financial Ratios *(continued)*

Explanation of Financial Ratios

1. *Current ratio* measures the liquidity of current assets and whether the entity has sufficient working capital to meet its short-term obligations. Profitable entities typically have higher current ratios, although this is not a hard-and-fast rule.

2. *Days of revenue in patient accounts receivable* measures the amount of time, on average, that receivables are outstanding. The shorter this time period, the better the cash flow situation.

3. *Days cash on hand* measures the number of days that expenses are covered by cash and short-term investments. A low value could signal the need for short-term borrowing to cover operating expenses.

4. *Average payment period* measures the amount of time, on average, that payables are outstanding. Cash flow improves as this period lengthens, but interest charges imposed by vendors for late payments should be considered.

5. *Operating margin* measures the proportion of operating revenue retained as income. If significant sums of money are received from sources other than operations (such as investments from endowments and contributions) and these funds are available for operations, they may be included in the ratio to measure operating margin. On the revenue side, operating margin can be influenced by the percentage of revenue derived from charge-based payers. On the cost side, effective cost-control measures will result in improvements (increases) in this ratio. This ratio can be used to measure the effectiveness of an entity's cost-control efforts.

6. *Return on equity* measures the increase in the entity's equity or profit per dollar invested in the entity. Because assets and other investments must be financed by either equity or debt and because no entity can continually sustain long-term growth with debt, equity growth is a key measure of an entity's long-term ability to replace and increase assets.

7. *Return on assets* measures the amount of "net income" (revenue and gains in excess of expenses and losses) earned per dollar of investment in assets. An entity's assets are its investments and must generate a return sufficient to replace themselves as necessary to maintain the entity's financial viability.

8. *Debt-to-equity or leverage ratio* measures the proportion of long-term debt to equity or net assets and reveals how dependent the entity is on long-term debt to finance assets. A high ratio together with substantial Medicare and Medicaid volumes could signal potential debt service difficulties because the reimbursement methods of some payers may not cover all costs.

9. *Debt service coverage ratio* measures how many debt service payments can be covered from operations. In the past, a 2:1 ratio was considered desirable. For a very large project, a somewhat lower level will still provide a reasonable level of comfort. A ratio below or not much greater than 1:1 raises concerns about the entity's future ability to cover debt and indicates that the entity's debt capacity is probably exhausted.

10. *Cash flow to total debt ratio* measures how many times total liabilities are covered from operations and is another measure of an entity's debt capacity and solvency.

11. *Average age of plant* measures the number of years of depreciation that have been expensed. It is a quick indicator of the need to replace or renovate the physical plant in the near future. If the average age indicates potential need for renovation but the debt service coverage ratio is close to 1:1, the entity may have a problem financing a needed project.

12. *Total asset turnover* measures the efficiency of capital investment. The more revenue that can be generated from an entity's investment in assets (that is, higher ratios), the more profitable the entity will be.

13. *Working capital turnover ratio* measures the ability of the entity to generate revenues from its investment in working capital. This ratio and similar ratios of turnover of asset categories (for example, inventory and receivables) can show trends in efficient or inefficient use and management of assets, particularly when compared over a period of several years.

The internal control structure is made up of three components: the control environment, accounting system, and control procedures. The *control environment* consists of the broad policies and procedures that provide the framework for the accounting system and control procedures. This framework reflects the level of control consciousness within an organization. The control environment is determined by the combination of the following elements:

- Management's philosophy and operating style
- The mechanisms established by management to create a framework for accounting systems and controls
- The external and internal influences on management that directly affect management's attitude toward financial reporting and controls

A health care organization's *accounting system* consists of the methods and records established to identify, assemble, analyze, classify, record, and report the organization's transactions. The accounting system should also maintain accountability for the organization's related assets and liabilities. An effective accounting system accurately records and reports all valid transactions.

A health care organization's *control procedures,* which are embedded throughout the organization's control environment and accounting system, provide reasonable assurance that specific objectives will be achieved. Generally, control procedures take the following forms:

- Proper authorization of transactions and activities
- Effective segregation of duties
- Design and use of appropriate documents and records
- Adequate safeguards over access to and use of assets and records
- Independent checks on performance
- Proper valuation of recorded amounts

Besides the preceding three traditional components of the internal control structure, health care entities may be subject to other audit and internal control requirements. For example, if an entity receives federal financial assistance such as research grants or matching funds, certain audit requirements may apply. Additional audit and internal control requirements will depend on the type of health care organization involved, the amount of financial assistance received, and the specific terms of the financial assistance award. These requirements may include "tests of controls" to evaluate the effectiveness of controls over an organization's compliance with certain laws and regulations applicable to the federal program funds. The board should ensure that effective controls are in place and that appropriate federal financial assistance audits are performed.

The establishment and monitoring of an effective internal control structure is critical to helping management and the board safeguard their health care organization's assets. However, certain control procedures may not be available to small health care organizations. For example, an organization with a small number of staff members may find it difficult or impossible to create segregation of duties or perform independent checks on performance. In these situations, a competent manager may function as a substitute for many of the formal control mechanisms previously listed. A manager of a small health care organization who assumes an active role in its day-to-day operations generally possesses a first-hand knowledge of all of the organization's business aspects. Such a manager would be able to effectively monitor and control business and would thus help to mitigate an absence of specific controls and a lack of segregation of duties. However, the board should recognize that it may be easy for management of a small health care organization to override whatever controls are in place.

Board members often ask, "How much internal control is enough?" At some point the cost of additional controls exceeds the benefits they provide, but identifying that point is not easy. The internal control structure should concentrate on *material errors* (unintentional misstatements) and *irregularities* (intentional misstatements). From a cost-and-benefit perspective, eliminating all errors and irregularities is impractical. Even if an internal control structure is well designed, it can be defeated by human errors, collusion among employees, or executive override. No internal control is a guarantee against errors and irregularities. The internal control structure can only provide reasonable assurance that errors and irregularities will be detected and/or prevented.

Internal Audit

Along with the independent auditors, a health care organization's internal auditors help board members meet their responsibilities for the financial reporting process. Traditionally, internal auditors are considered to be control specialists, and their role is to study, evaluate, and test the internal control structure. When internal auditors perform these duties, they perform a special control function for the board. They are not a part of internal accounting control in the same manner as an individual who verifies the accuracy of billings; they represent a higher level of control that determines whether the system is functioning. Internal auditors are able to provide the board with an independent and objective view that is difficult for management to provide. As a result, their assurances go a long way toward helping the board fulfill its responsibilities.

Some boards ask internal auditors to perform activities that go beyond their previously described traditional roles. One of these activities might be to review administrative controls in such areas as personnel management, information systems, budgeting, cost management, and materials management. Reviewing controls in these areas can help ensure that established policies are followed, and frequently these reviews generate ideas for improving an organization's efficiency.

If internal auditors are to function effectively, their work must be carefully planned. Although internal auditors are sometimes used as extra hands to assist management in special projects, these projects should not override the auditors' primary responsibility to the auditing program. If the internal audit function is to help management and the board fulfill their monitoring responsibilities, a comprehensive auditing program should be developed that will allow internal auditors to systematically review all important aspects of internal control on a planned basis. The board and management must ensure that the internal audit function has qualified personnel who have been given enough training and time to complete their planned program of internal audits.

References

1. Healthcare Financial Management Association. Principles and Practices Board Statement No. 15, "Valuation and Financial Statement Presentation of Charity Service and Bad Debts by Institutional Healthcare Providers."

2. American Institute of Certified Public Accountants. *Audit and Accounting Guide: Audits of Providers of Health Care Services.* Chicago: Commerce Clearing House, 1993.

3. American Institute of Certified Public Accountants. Statement of Auditing Standards No. 55, "Consideration of the Internal Control Structure in a Financial Statement Audit."

Additional Books of Interest

Hospital-Physician Integration: Strategies for Success

by Terence M. Murphy and C. Thompson Hardy
published in cooperation with the New England Health Care Assembly

This book is a must-read for any hospital or physician group considering exploring integration options.

Hospital-Physician Integration provides an in-depth discussion of the major issues that are crucial to the process of integrating health care delivery systems. It focuses on the affiliation of existing organizations and presents the issues both through an analysis of the process as well as the presentation of seven detailed case studies.

Catalog No. E99-145159 (must be included when ordering)
1994. 237 pages, 54 figures, 12 tables.
$57.50 (AHA members, $46.00)

The Art of Fund-Raising:
What Every Health Care Trustee Needs to Know

by Edward Hugh Bovich, Edward Philip Bovich, Ph.D.,
and John Patrick Bovich, J.D.

This unique book
- helps institutions find new financial resources through charitable donations
- describes the trustee's role and responsibility in fund-raising
- explains how to encourage contributions based on the donor's motivations for giving
- presents 10 principles of good fund-raising
- discusses four approaches to raising funds
- illustrates successful strategies with real-life examples

Catalog No. E99-196128 (must be included when ordering)
1994. 199 pages, 3 figures, 3 tables.
$35.00 (AHA members, $28.00)

To order, call TOLL FREE
800-AHA-2626.

DATE DUE			
AUG 21 95			
10-17-95			
FEB 26 96			
FEB 17 1997			
APR 2 1 1997			
MAY 30 2009			